The Cryptic Pregnancy Files the doctors are lying to you!
Neo Brown

Copyright 2022: A.E.L Burrowes

DISCLAIMER: This book is designed to provide information. It is sold with the understanding that the author & the publisher are not engaged to render any type of psychological, medical, legal, or any other professional advice. This book is not meant to be used, nor should it be used, to diagnose or treat any medical condition. For diagnosis or treatment of any medical problem, consult your own physician. The publisher & author are not responsible for any specific health or allergy needs that may require medical supervision and are not liable for any damages or negative consequences from any treatment, action, application, or preparation to any person reading or following the information in this book. The content of each chapter is the sole expression & opinion of the author. The publisher & the individual author shall not be liable for any physical, psychological, emotional, financial, or any commercial damages, including, but not limited to, special, incidental, consequential or other damages.

ABOUT THE AUTHOR

Neo Brown is a Medical Researcher & Cryptic Pregnancy Pioneer. She began the first online conversation about a Cryptic Pregnancy in her yahoo group Pregnant but Negative Tests over a decade ago. She has a degree in Biochemistry & read some Theology at Spurgeon's College London. She has written two books.

And you shall know the truth & the truth shall set you free. John 8 v32

My motto is: believe what you like as ether way I'm good.

This book is dedicated to Golden.
Thank you for listening back in the day.

Table of content

Chapter one the problem

Chapter two: Important Spiritual & Gnostic Truths

Chapter three: Why a woman's cycle often continues during a CP

Chapter four: CP & Divine birth: Many CP children are self-conceived

Chapter five: How to be pregnant with a CP & look & live like you're not

Chapter six: Case studies of CP women who had healthy CP babies

Chapter seven: How to fix a CP

Chapter eight: The dangers of ignoring a CP

Chapter nine: The fibroid, dermoid cyst & pregnancy of unknown location lie

Chapter ten: How to deal with medical professionals during a CP

Bibliography

1.
The Problem

Here in 2022 women all over the world in every race & culture are experiencing what has been labelled A CRYPTIC PREGNANCY. Social media, especially Facebook is littered with thousands of women and hundreds of groups trying and failing to understand this often-devastating female Phenomenon.

So, what is a Cryptic Pregnancy exactly?

Well, it's not what wiki would lead you to believe but then, when does wiki ever tell The Truth? Answers on a postcard might be nice.

Cryptic pregnancies have been called hidden pregnancies historically in non-western countries.

The word cryptic means hidden or obscure. It is my purpose with this book to reveal the Truths that have been hidden for so long about a cryptic pregnancy.

In my personal experience of studying a cryptic pregnancy for over ten years, going through one myself more than once, giving birth to healthy CP babies & from talking to hundreds of women who have been through a cryptic pregnancy it is:

A: NOT a phantom pregnancy. A phantom or delusional pregnancy is something the medical cartel (Aka most medical professionals.) call a cryptic pregnancy. This is because most of them are blind fools & robots & do not possess the spiritual capability to expand their mental or spiritual awareness, or even the simple ability to apply basic common sense & look for a fetal heartbeat.

B. A cryptic pregnancy or CP is not a woman who doesn't know she's pregnant until she gives birth. Although for a few lucky CP women this can be a happy conclusion to a hellish nightmare.

But this is not the majority.

A cryptic pregnancy is a frightening yet physical situation where a woman is actually pregnant BUT has ether completely negative or faint positive pregnancy tests. The faint positives are always ignored & explained away by the medical cartel (medical professionals.) Who do very little, if anything to investigate despite the pleading & obvious distress of the patient.

How do we know a woman is ACTUALLY pregnant during a CP?

The answer is quite simple yet almost completely out of the logical reach of most of the medical cartel. Having a CP is like being in the film The Lazarus project. The doctors are telling you one thing, but the opposite is true. But I am here to tell you that you CAN prove your pregnancy.

Let me take you back.

Up until the mid-80s in the UK most GPs used a stethoscope to help confirm pregnancy. Doctors used common sense & logic if a woman felt pregnant, but tests were negative. Sadly, these days most medical students are not taught these basic skills. They are taught to ONLY rely upon tests & hard facts.

My own mother's pregnancy with me was confirmed with a stethoscope & her pulse being taken. My mother had felt pregnant, missed at least four cycles & had been feeling sick but couldn't get a positive on a home pregnancy test.

According to her the GP took her pulse, whilst using his stethoscope on her slightly swollen belly & confirmed her pregnancy.

He didn't even bother to do another pregnancy test!

Why? Because doctors knew then as they should know now the golden rule of a cryptic pregnancy is that:

No human being alive has two SEPARATE heartbeats inside of one body.

My mother's GP therefore understood that because he found a heartbeat inside her belly that was DIFFERENT & therefore SEPARATE from her own heartbeat, the heartbeat he found by simply taking her pulse, (from her radial artery in her wrist.) she was actually pregnant.

Despite her negative pregnancy tests.

I am of course the result of that cryptic pregnancy.

Now although many women do continue a cycle during a CP it should change by becoming shorter or lighter. You might even miss a few.

The high dose hook effect has been discussed in medical journals & peer reviewed papers for many years & you can find these easily online.

I have found that at least 50% of CP women are suffering from the high dose hook effect.

The high dose hook effect happens when your body produces too MUCH HCG & the pregnancy test can't handle it, so it reads NEGATIVE.

These are FALSE negative pregnancy tests.

If you are showing the sign & symptoms of pregnancy your doctor should be willing to order a pregnancy blood test that tests for the high dose hook effect.
In the lab water is added to your blood sample by titration. This dilutes your pregnancy blood sample very slowly until the pregnancy test turns positive for pregnancy.

You can also dilute your urine sample at home to try this. Start with the ratio of adding one part water to one part urine then increase the water ratio until you see a positive pregnancy test.

It's best to try this with pregnancy test strips as they are not too expensive.

This has worked for many CP women I know.

If you think you are having a CP & have never had a positive pregnancy test (you should be testing at least once a week throughout your CP.) try diluting your urine sample as described above to see if your negatives are false negatives, due to the high dose hook effect.

Sadly, even if you get several positive pregnancy tests this way most doctors will dismiss it. Why?

Because for at least the last twenty years medical schools have not been teaching students logical & deductive thinking. As a result, most doctors cannot think creatively so if your pregnancy test at the doctor's office is negative, like a silly robot he is programmed mentally to NOT question that test because he has been brain washed, I mean taught in medical school that his medical tests are the only kind of truth that exist on planet earth.

Most women are diagnosed with polycystic ovary syndrome during a CP but be INCREDIBLY careful of this diagnosis. Why?

Well, a doctor has got to eat right?

Often when the medical cartel can't figure something out or want to blatantly hide the truth about a situation (I will prove in later chapters that many doctors have lied & covered up evidence when a woman is actually pregnant during a CP. I know women who have sued doctors for these cover ups.) they label you with a syndrome. A syndrome isn't really an illness or a diagnosis it's a collection of indefinite symptoms.

According to the dictionary a syndrome is, "a group of symptoms which consistently occur together." So, it's vague on purpose. Some of the symptoms of PCOS are the same as a CP: irregular periods or no periods at all, (well make up your mind doc it's ether one or the other surely?) not being able to conceive, (of course you can't conceive if you are already pregnant with a CP baby.) & Weight gain. (Definitely part of a CP to an extent because women having a CP are actually pregnant & do pregnant women gain weight? Yes.)

Hair growth on the face or chest is also apparently a symptom of PCOS.

True story, when I was pregnant with my son's, I always had one or two stay hairs grow on my chest. It really freaked me out but my GP doctor at the time told me it was quite common & just from the extra male hormone in my body from being pregnant with a boy. I know other non-CP women who have had this during their pregnancy with a boy. The hairs thankfully never came back after I had my sons.

So, you see, PCOS definitely has symptoms that fit with a CP. It's a great little non disease the doctors just love to label CP women with because if her pregnancy tests are negative a doctor will NEVER try & investigate the possibility of pregnancy further.

One symptom that does NOT fit with PCOS is fetal movement. If you are truly having a CP as in, you are REALLY pregnant, but your pregnancy tests are falsely negative you will be able to feel the baby move from around five months CP. As the months progress you should at times feel the kind of movement that can make you jump. I have seen videos of CP women online where you can literally see a baby's FOOT poke out of the CP woman's belly it's kicking so hard, but they don't think they are pregnant at all because their doctor has told them, "Oh that's just gas! Your pregnancy tests are negative, so you are NOT PREGNANT. Gas however often develops feet & can kick you really hard & it might seem like a baby, but because your tests are negative IT'S NOT."

So, most CP women believe the great white coat as who are we mere mortals to go against the great high priest of the medical cartel, I mean the doctors diagnosis?

Please. You really have to start thinking for yourself during a CP if you want the best outcome. Never suspend your common sense & accept what any doctor, midwife or medical professionals tell you. Do your own research, it's your life not theirs & you only get one.

If you are awake this should already be very obvious to you.

The other huge symptom that does not fit with PCOS is hearing a baby's heartbeat on a fetal Doppler whilst USING A FINGER PLUSE to detect your own heartbeat at the same time.

Can you test this theory yourself?

Yes, you can. Buy a fetal doppler & a finger pulse & follow the instructions of both.
Use the finger pulse on your finger at the same time you use the doppler to hear the baby's heartbeat in your belly.

An adult resting heart rate will be around 60bpm to 90bpm a baby's 120 to 170bpm.

You will often hear very loud MOVEMENT from your belly & even feel it kick at the doppler. This is the baby. Babies tend to hate dopplers, just ask any decant midwife, so they move to try & get away from it.

I am sorry but bowels DO NOT MOVE because they haven't got arms & legs. This is a favourite stupid lie the medical cartel will try & tell you if you tell them, you have used a doppler & heard a lot of movement.

There are a lot of paid shills & disinformation agents on Facebook & YouTube whose job it is to cover up CP Truth & confuse it. They are useless robots, have no spirit or soul with in them & you can detect this from their dead eyes & dead Energy on screen.

They try & use the doppler alone when you need a finger pulse to confirm, on their non pregnant belly to prove that bowls have heartbeats of over 120bpm. This is of course a lie.

The doppler barley register any number & the noises you hear on these videos are only heard because they are breathing very heavily on purpose to create sound or because they are moving the probe too much. You have to keep the probe really still once you have found the baby's heartbeat & the baby's heart rate numbers come up & do not disappear.

As a side note, I have heard recently about strange witch doctor types trying to give women who are desperate for a child a CP. This is so illogical I can hardly comprehend it.
Exactly how unintelligent do you have to be in order to swallow this lie? But some do apparently.

No kind of fertility treatment can GIVE you a CP & dear God WHY WOULD ANYONE IN THEIR RIGHT MIND WANT ONE? A CP is one of the worst things a woman will ever go through.

Most women have a very normal pregnancy as a result of fertility treatment & their pregnancy tests are clearly positive from the first day of a missed cycle if not before.

NEVER take any medicine or herbs to help turn your CP normal as this is also a SCAM. Only you can turn your CP normal. I will explain how in chapter seven.

NEVER take anything to try & induce CP. CP babies often grow at different rates to normal babies & often stop growing only to start again. (Also explained in chapter seven.) So doing so can & has resulted in the sad loss of a CP baby.

I won't waste my brain power on saying any more than this about these people but again, as a True spiritual Being you have the power to be able to read their dead negative Energy when you watch them speak on YouTube too so be your own judge & learn how to read Energy or the vibe of these women. It only takes a little practice.

These shills never use a FINGER PULSE to confirm their own heartbeat whilst using the doppler on these CP vlogs so that is a huge indication that they have no idea what they are talking about. You need to use the finger plus as well as the doppler to confirm that a CP is a True pregnancy.

Just keep practising with the doppler & the finger pulse. Your pulse or heartbeat will be between 60 to 90bpm a baby's is 120 to 170bpm as I have said.

Once you have found these two separate heartbeats you know you are pregnant. It doesn't matter how long you have been pregnant, how negative your pregnancy tests are whether you continue to have a cycle or not or what the doctors say.
The two separate heartbeats are the hardcore evidence that prove a woman is actually pregnant during a CP, but doctors choose to ignore this fact. Finding a second heartbeat in a woman would confirm pregnancy forty years ago so why not now?

> But the Truth is the Truth. Are you bold enough to accept it?

2.
Important spiritual & Gnostic truths

In this book I will reveal to you the things not one doctor, scientists, pastor, priest, researcher, or anyone from the medical profession have been able to understand & reveal about what a cryptic pregnancy really is, how to prove it, how to LIVE with it whilst keeping slim so it doesn't ruin or control your life and lastly, but perhaps most importantly:
how to turn a CP into a normal pregnancy.

Who I am isn't important, the most important thing to ask yourself is:
Do these Truths actually work & will they help to ease & relieve the suffering CP women & their family's go through every second of every day all over the world?

I believe that they will. These Truths worked for me & many other CP women who I have shared them with so please do your best to read this book with an open mind & heart.

Firstly, please understand that suffering is NOT from God.

Just think about it, why would a loving parent punish a child continually just to teach it a lesson?

Would you treat your own children this way? Of course not!

Then why oh, why do we pretend that trials & suffering, such as going through a CP, a situation where a woman is REALLY pregnant but because her pregnancy tests are negative nobody in the medical cartel will believe or help her, is a test sent from a loving God?

It's in the bible you say. Well, the bible has many contradictory versions & has been tampered with & changed relentlessly over the last three thousand years by evil people.

This might be ridiculously hard to accept if you grew up as a Christian like I did but the logic of these words are facts that often only a thinking person can understand.

Once we see that a CP is not a trial or a test from a loving God, but an unwanted circumstance put on some women by evil (the devil, lucifer Satan or whatever you personally name it.) then we will begin to realise that this is a WAR & your very life plus the life of your unborn CP baby could be at stake. A CP is not a safe happy-clappy time where you can ignore the doctors non confirmation & walk around with a huge pregnant belly for years as your life falls apart around you.

It is a war.

Have you ever wondered why there are some people around who are so hard to get alone with & often cause much pain & upset to others?
Violent or abusive partners are a perfect example. No matter how often they promise to change or even seek help they never seem to be able to.
The emotional, mental & often physical pain they put their abused partners & children through is never endings.

Today these people are often called sociopaths, narcissists or even psychopaths.

The Jesus of the bible would have called them demons. Yes,
that's right I said demons.

Jesus didn't fight ghosts in the air as the church & lots of twisted scripture would have you believe.

He fought human beings who were not possessed by devils but WERE devils walking in flesh.

This is why these people never respond to love, kindness, or empathy. They do not possess the ability to do so. You cannot change them with enough love.

Ever.

You see, according to the original Gnostics & Gnostic texts, some of which are in the bible (but you need the Nous or spiritual knowing within you to understand them.) there are two creations. So, there are two types of humans walking the earth today.

Because on this earth not all humans are equal spiritually.
It's very evident as most people hate the idea of God & Truth. We have all met these people at work, school & socially. Some are even in our family.

No, you are not supposed to turn the other cheek & keep letting devils in human suits drain your energy & abuse you. You must stay AWAY from these people. Specially if you are having a CP.

We have all heard of a fake handbag or a fake watch. They look terribly similar to the real thing, but they are completely fake!

So, it is with demons & robotic consciousness humans. They can be any race & any gender. They look like humans & even act like humans most of the time, but they are not human. They are FAKE humans.
REAL humans have a divine consciousness, are moral & have a natural awareness & love for Truth.

They hate to argue or cause upset. They want peace & are often naturally happy, calm & peaceful.

According to Ancient Gnostic Truth these are the True children of the one True God the Absolute.
The fake humans or demons are of their father the devil, or Jehovah the evil God of the Old Testament who loved blood sacrifice. He created them to drain & destroy the children of the Absolute or The Light.

Do you have pets? Look at your beloved pets or look on TikTok or IG & watch reels of cute pets.
Now answer me this:

What kind of god would want anyone to sacrifice or kill their beautiful pet just because he wanted a blood sacrifice that day?

It's evil & illogical yet most who grew up with a form of Christianity bought into this lie. I myself was guilty of believing for many years that the god of the Old Testament was the One True God but no he is an error & an imposter.

Only the devil or Jehovah the fake god of the Old Testament, the demiurge could demand such evil.

Just think about it for a moment. Use your own inner mind not your pastors.

A REAL human or True Being as they are often referred to, have a lot of spiritual Energy with in them. The fake humans or demons' sole purpose in life whether they know it or not, is to drain the Real human of this Energy. Like a spiritual vampire, this is how it survives.

Have you ever seen a person who seems to look pleased with themselves when they cause arguments or upset people? That person is a perfect example of a fake demonic human.

As True Beings you now have the power to read the Energy of these people so you can stay away from them & not date or marry them. If you are already in a relationship with one, ask God to help you get out of it. The separation of Light from darkness, the wheat from the tares, the True Being

from non-True Being is well underway in this generation & if you are paired with a fake human or demon, you will be given the wisdom & strength to go your separate ways. If you love Truth & the One True God more than anything you will be willing & able to break away from them sooner rather than later. The Light will make a way & show you how.
We are in the end times & this is particularly important for your spiritual health & survival.

I haven't got time to go into more Gnostic Truth here but the best books on these important spiritual facts are any books or articles by Dr. Joseph Chiappalone who is both a medical & metaphysic

doctor. I have all of his books, but Essential Gnostic Truth is one of my favourites. His books are on eBay worldwide & his articles can be found at rense.com.

They are priceless yet not expensive so if you can get a copy of any of his books you will be extremely blessed & glad that you did.

Another brilliant book that might be hard to buy but is available online in pdf form is JEHOVAH UNMASKED! By Nathaniel J Merritt. This book really helped me to wake up to basic spiritual Gnostic Truths.

So why is this information so important for women going through a CP?

Talking to CP women from all over the world for the last ten years I have noticed that many of them are True Beings & real humans created by the Absolute. They have a real love for Truth & God & I can just read it in their Energy from talking to them.

This is key because it shows that a CP is partly a spiritual ATTACK on most CP women. This is not God attacking you but Jehovah the evil demiurge as Plato called it or the evil god of this world as Jesus called it.

Because you are a True Being your spiritual Energy is needed in this evil dimension, so the suffering & heartache caused by a CP is supposed to drain & destroy you spiritually.

You must understand this but do not fear because the Truth in this book will help to set you & your baby free from a CP.

Everything in this world is about Energy. Some call its life force, chi, or prana.

The loss of vital Energy due to a CP is partly why some CP women are pregnant for years. No, you won't believe it unless it happens to you & even then you will find it hard to believe but if you have a fetal doppler & a finger pulse you can prove it to yourself at least as I explained in chapter one.

The loss of Energy during a CP is a trap as it is a vicious circle. You feel pregnant but your tests are negative. You seek help from doctors. They tell you you're not pregnant as your tests are negative but will not investigate further. If they do investigate further WHATEVER they find, & the doctor

often actually SEES a baby on your scan, they cannot tell you that you ARE pregnant purely BECAUSE your tests are negative because doing so could threaten their very career.

Yes, the days are very evil & Truth is stranger than fiction. I have heard this from many CP women & seen their scan reports over the years & it is clear from most that there is a baby on the scan.

I saw a baby of at least six months gestation on a scan during my pregnancy with one of my CP children, but the doctor said there was nothing there at all. He lied to my face, but I had the last Laugh.
As a CP woman gets no help from the medical cartel, she gets more stressed & depressed. This loss of vital Energy just prolongs her CP.
Some CP women have even tragically taken their own lives because of all of this.

The only people to blame are the doctors & the medical cartel for not putting aside their precious tests for a second & for not using basic logic & listening for a fetal heartbeat to confirm pregnancy as they did thirty or forty years ago.

Many doctors (most but not all.) are evil fake humans & demons so it is easy for them to lie to a CP woman sadly.

But You CAN break the awful cycle of a CP. There are no guarantees in this life but the knowledge of why the cycle happens & how to break it are in this book.

3.
Why her cycle continues

As females we all dread the awful witch who comes knocking every month. Pregnancy is usually a welcome nine months of cycle free living but for a CP woman the cycle often doesn't stop. It can be lighter and or shorter, but it continues.

Well let's back up a bit & ask a valid question:

Do all healthy women of childbearing age bleed every month?

Let's not get it twisted. Hands up who actually likes having a cycle? Nobody does! It's annoying & painful & UNHEALTHY.

Why? Because you are BLEEDING!

Now before you close this book & tell me you know how biology works just think:

What if MEN bled every month? Every doctor alive would put everything into stopping it!

Yet women are expected to carry on as normal whilst we are bleeding for four to seven days a month.
No wonder many women are depressed & exhausted most of the time. During a monthly cycle we lose vital blood & fluid. It's even worse if you are going through a CP because the blood loss isn't good for you or the baby.

Again, most of us have swallowed the Christian lie from genesis 3 v13 NKJV:
"To the woman he said: I will greatly multiply your sorrow and your conception; in pain you shall bring forth children."

Obviously, this was spoken by the evil god of the Old Testament, the demiurge who according to Gnostics rebelled against the Absolute The One True God, created earth, trapped True Beings in these bodies of flesh & just because he felt like it & amongst other things, cursed women to bleed each month & have pain in childbirth.

& You want to worship this guy?!

I'm so glad so many are waking up & leaving the Christian church in droves all over the world. If you love the Truth, you will be led by the Nous within you. You do not need a church or a pastor to be close to God.

So please understand that the Supreme Truth, Allah, Jesus, shiva, the Great Spirit, the Absolute or whatever you call IT did NOT say that a woman most bleed or suffer every month in order to have children.

So why are we accepting this awful monthly suffering CP or not?

Did you know that female animal mammals both domesticated & in the wild do NOT bleed each month, yet they have lots of healthy offspring?

Again, religion & science have tricked woman kind into accepting this huge lie.

One of my favourite books on this subject is: the Psychological Enigma of woman: The Mystery of Menstruation by Dr. Raymond w. Bernard.

On page 123 he says, ". in ancient times the women of India did not menstruate & considered menstruation a crime."

In the next paragraph he describes that there are parts of Brazil where women have NEVER had a cycle or monthly bleed and YET they have had lots of healthy children.

Even the bible described a woman's monthly cycle as a sickness in lev 15: 33.
They have tried to cover up the word sickness & it's changed in newer bible version but the literal standard version & the American standard version say, "and of her who is sick with her impurity…is unclean."
There is a lot of Gnostic Truth in the bible, but you need the spiritual eyes to see what is real & what is not.

Now why would the ancient text of Leviticus call a cycle both a sickness & an impurity?

Because it is BOTH a sickness & can be the result of impurity.

Come on now think about it.

Stay with me for a moment & I will make this Truth as plain as day.

In the book Dr Raymond W. Bernard has a lot to say about how exactly a woman can stop her monthly cycle since it is of course a sickness or an illness & should be seen by any thinking person by now to be as such, despite what society & most doctors will tell you.

He talks about many wise doctors who succeeded in helping women ether completely stop their cycle each month or reduce it to almost nothing.

The most interesting thing he ultimately said helped to stop the witch from arriving each month was to greatly reduce sexual activity.

An unpopular opinion to most & quite odd to say the least as many women are married or in relationships.

My concern however in only with CP women.

Sex is obviously not impure or wrong in a decant relationship unless you are a True Being or Real human & your sexual partner is a demon or a fake human.

As Doctor Joseph Chiappalone points out in his brilliant book Journey into the World of Metaphysics volume one, sex between a True Being & a demon or fake human (remember all humans may look similar but it is the consciousness WITHIN that makes a human ether a True Being or a demon.) always results in a huge loss of positive spiritual Energy or Life force for the True Being & the accumulation of negative polluting Energy from the demon or fake human.

This is the single prefect reason to ALWAYS go with your gut when choosing a partner.

If something feels off or you don't vibe with them do not get involved.

As a True Being your spirit or higher self will make you feel uneasy, agitated, or ill if you try & get it on with a demon or a fake human. Your lack of sex drive is not the problem mainstream media would have you believe it is. It's a protection mechanism employed by The Light to stop you from sleeping with someone who is a danger to your spiritual wellbeing. Remember you can't tell if a guy is a demon just by looking at him. You need to be able to read Energy & even if you do have this gift it needs to be developed.

You will have to be ether drunk or able to ignore your gut instinct completely if you want to date or hook up with a fake human or demon. Nether situation is recommended for obvious reasons.

ENERGY OR LIFE FORCE LOSS is the main reason CP women continue to have a cycle throughout a CP.

No, it's not just having sex with a fake human, it's the Energy loss she experiences from the vicious circle that is a CP:

she feels pregnant, her pregnancy tests are negative, doctors won't help BECAUSE her tests are negative, rinse & repeat.

The pain & suffering in everyday life because of this situation causes a HIGE amounts of Energy loss.

If her partner is ALSO a demon or fake human whilst she is a True Being the Energy loss is catastrophic partly due to sex, so of course her monthly cycle continues because continued bleeding each month during a CP is due ultimately, to spiritual pollution & what better way to pollute than through sex?

I have tested this theory with one of my own CP pregnancies by ending a relationship with a definite demon (I was always careful to remain slim during my CPs, so I never allowed myself to look pregnant until after the pregnancy was confirmed.) & Becoming celibate & not dating anyone & definitely not hooking up with any non-True Being & my cycle stopped in a matter of months.

I know of other CP women who have been led to leave lovers or partners who were of the wrong consciousness & their cycles also stopped within months of the split too.

Throughout this book I will present case studies of real-life situations from CP women around the world who have told me their stories to illustrate these facts. I will also reveal some of my own CP story. However, names will be changed to protect our privacy.

In light of this meet Ella.

Ella is thirty-eight, a part time teacher & already a mother to an eighteen-year-old who is in full time education & lives on campus.

Because of loneliness & against her better judgment she begins dating Mike who was a successful author but drinks too much. Ella only ever drinks socially once or twice a month.

Since her son left home, she agreed to let her new partner move in. Big mistake.

Soon she feels pregnant & of course she knows how it feels to be pregnant. She takes lots of pregnancy tests, but they are all negative. Despite this her belly begins to grow in line with the pregnancy.

She is having a cryptic pregnancy & yes you guessed it, her GP would not help her or use common sense & listen for a fetal heartbeat as her tests are negative. Instead, he threatens her (now you know why I call them the medical cartel.) & Says she will be forced to see the mental health team if she doesn't stop insisting, she is pregnant with negative tests.

So, she pays for a private scan. The tech says that she does see something but as her pregnancy tests are negative, she is told it could be a fibroid so she should go back to her GP. Ella isn't stupid. She's very intuitive & knows she is pregnant despite the negative tests. She knows that she doesn't have a fibroid (after a scan a CP woman is often told she has a fibroid. I have seen much evidence even during my own CPs to suggest that what doctors often call a fibroid is actually a live healthy CP baby but because her HCG tests are negative the foetus is labelled as a fibroid. More on this in chapter nine.)

Her cycle doesn't stop but reduces from six days of bleeding to three.

Ella is wise enough NOT to tell Mike about her CP. She wears baggy clothes & tries to watch what she eats as who wants to LOOK pregnant with negative tests & therefore no confirmation?

His drinking increases as his new book doesn't get published & worse, she has to hide all of her spiritual books because Mike is not just an atheist, he hates any mention or sight of things remotely spiritual. (Mike has a demonic consciousness.)

Mike is emotionally manipulative & abusive so finally Ella finds the strength to kick him out of her house.

Now she is really alone. No partner, her son away at uni & now a CP pregnancy. She can't even consider an abortion as of course without a positive pregnancy test she thinks she can't have one.

At this point Ella reached out to me in me secrete Facebook group called The Cryptic Pregnancy Files.

I explained my findings about stopping her monthly cycle & how to eat & exercise to stay slim during her CP until her tests turn normal. I also shared with Ella the Gnostic Truths in chapter two.

Being a True Being & having always felt close to God in her own way my words strongly resonated with her.

Soon she makes her home her own again & puts her spiritual books back on the shelf. She had a lot of health problems due to her CP (high blood pressure & depression.) but she buys a puppy & this helps to relieve her loneliness & depression greatly.

She obviously wasn't sleeping with Mike since the split & although she still felt pregnant as was still going through a CP, she no longer LOOKED pregnant after taking my advice.

She did not however look for a new relationship.

Three months after her split with Mike her cycle stopped completely. At thirty-eight this is too early for menopause as this happens to most women around the age of fifty.

Ella soon has faint positive pregnancy tests & was grateful for this progress as she had never had a positive test during her CP when Mike was around.

She is hopeful for the future & positive about the real possibility of bringing up her baby alone.

So, you see from Ella's CP case study that once she ended her abusive relationship & spent more time on herself her cycle stopped & her tests began to turn positive. This was huge.

The vital life force she needed to help to turn her CP into a normal pregnancy was no longer being lost through sex with Mike, an abusive alcoholic who was also a demonic consciousness human.

You must protect your Energy & life force as doing this is part of the KEY to turning a CP into a normal pregnancy.

Why wasn't Ella sad that she would have to bring up the baby alone without Mike the father?
Some people think any father is better for a child than no father at all specially for financial reasons. Mike was not in fact the father of Ella's CP baby although she was sleeping with him at the time of conception. Yes, you read that right. How can that be possible? In the next chapter all will be revealed.

4.
CP & divine birth

MANY CP CHILDREN ARE SELF CONCEIVED

We've all heard stories of virgin & divine births. Christianity insists that Mary was the only woman to have ever had one, but the bible has been twisted over centuries by the kind of men who needed the truth about SOME women to be kept hidden.

The Truth is that some women today can self-conceive & no they do not have to be virgins to do so. It is also true that most CP pregnancies are actually self-conceived.

This is partly why the tests remain negative & the pregnancy lasts for so long because a baby who only has the genetics of its mother must produce HCG differently. However, through epigenetics, which is gene or DNA expression the child can look like it's father. This will be covered in depth in The Cryptic Pregnancy Files volume two.

It's my opinion that only female True Beings or Real humans (please see chapter two for an explanation of this.) can self-conceive or conceive by parthenogenesis. They may have DIFFERENT DNA so their physical abilities may be enhanced through their increased inherent spiritual ability to connect with the One True God.

I am not talking about religion here. Most people who are close to God wouldn't set foot inside of a church because all religions have twisted the Truth about The One True God on purpose to trap True Beings & to keep them from real Gnostic Truth.

Women who are fake humans or demons rarely possess the spiritual components needed for self-conception to occur, or for the foetus to grow into a healthy full term CP baby.

If they did MOST women today would be having a CP & more would have to be done to investigate it.

There is a huge cover up regarding a CP & all by design. I have spoken to many CP women who have shown me credible evidence that their babies for example are clearly seen on scans, even the tech or doctors surprise & shock have been recorded by them. CP babies can be clearly seen on X-rays, yet the CP mother is LIED to again & again by the medical cartel.

Why the cover up? Because if there are some women who can self-conceive it means there are two types of women on earth today PHYSICALLY.

This is not about colour or race. CP women are from all races but if the consciousness within a woman is that of a True Being she has more chance of self-conception & the powers that be / the illuminati/ the elite whatever you want to call them, must try & hide this.

All humans are equal & should always have equal rights & be treated equally on this earth.

But all humans are not equal ontologically or spiritually.

This should be obvious just from everyday life.

I personally have had huge physical & personal opposition in the last ten years whilst I have been researching for this book.

This is no coincidence.

Now there are no absolutes in this dimension so the demiurge MAY allow some of his fake human women to selfconceive or have a CP to add confusion as there is always an exception to a rule, but I have read books & articles by women who know self-conception still occurs today but being of a demonic nature try crazy stupid things to try & self-conceive themselves.

From squatting over herbs to strange sexual practices.

Please understand that self-conception has NOTHING to do with sex so even if you were having sex with your partner at the time of your CP conception, he is not the biological father. YOUR own body enabled conception & I will prove this scientifically not just metaphysically.

The ancients,' knowing self-conception was possible, tried all sorts of things to achieve it.
Many believed lying out in the sun could make you self-conceive but if that were the case, almost every woman who goes on a beach holiday each year would end up pregnant & most, without having had sex & is this really the case? Of course not.

In the interesting book Primitive Paternity by E S Hartland, the Anthropologist lists many of the strange practice's women all over the world did & would still do today no doubt if they thought for a second, they could really selfconceive. From drinking water from a particular river to eating a special stew.

Whilst we might smile at this, female True Beings who can & do self-conceive, & again these pregnancies are usually CP or hidden pregnancies, know deep down that they do not have to do anything half as crude to achieve it.

It takes zero effort if you have this ability. However, what you are spiritually is important.

In fact, you may do it without being aware of it since the original word conception literally means to conceive an idea.

Dr Raymond w. Bernard explains it simply & eloquently in The Mysteries Of Reproduction, "In 1852, just before the present theory of epigenesis became popular and accepted by the medical profession, john B Newman, M.D, published a book, still found in medical libraries, 'The Philosophy of Generation,' in this book he expresses that conception is effected not by the passage of semen into the uterus, and then to the egg, but by an impression (radiation or power from the Absolute?) upon the nervous system of the female. This impression travels up to the brain from where, instantly radiating to every part of the body, it falls on the ovaries, and acts on the maturing germs ready to receive it, giving the impressionable egg the governing influences, which must continue its existence. The outer coat of the germ bursts, and the finger like extremities of the Fallopian tube grasp it and convey it to the womb." Words in brackets mine.

Everything in science today stems from the relativity new philosophy of materialism so could it be that the few women on the planet today who are closer to the Spiritual maintain this rare ability to self-conceive?

In my experience all CP women who believed they self-conceived were remarkably close to The Truth, The Light, to God, Jesus, Allah, Shiva, Buddha, The Great Spirit or the Absolute, from Childhood.

In the New Testament Apocrypha Mary, the mother of Jesus was dedicated to the temple from childhood & could often be found talking & singing to God in the temple. Of course, she went on to self-conceive Jesus.

If you grew up with a thirst or huge interest in God & spent a lot of time reading about him to get to know him & Truth, then this could be you.

It takes no effort to be close to God despite what religion tells you. You just follow your passion & you just ARE.

Me & my best friend at children's church used to laugh at the people who said, "let's bow our heads & pray." Or "I got up early & prayed from 6am to 7am today bless God!"

We thought it was funny because we didn't use words like pray to talk to God, we just talked to him! Our connection with God was as real & as natural as breathing & completely free from religion even in childhood.

People talk about the God gene. I'm sure the God gene & CP women who self-conceive are directly related.

A bible verse that might help understanding is John 15v 5, "I am the vine; you are the branches. If you abide in me & I in you, you will bear much fruit …"

This verse will speak to those women who have this rare ability & of course there is no sex whatsoever involved in this kind of conception.

As it stands many CP women did NOT have sex at the time of their CP conception or their tubes were tied.
I have read accounts of A&E doctors who have treated women coming in complaining of extreme abdominal pain. These women were found to be in labour, but they swore blind to the doctors that they NEVER HAD SEX! Obviously, most doctors are blind robots, so they didn't believe these women for a second but in light of what I have just revealed, these women were almost certainly telling the truth because they were having a CP, had self-conceived & just didn't know it.

You don't have to consciously do anything to self-conceive IF you have this ability, your higher self or the One True God might show you that you will or have self-conceived, but you do not have to do anything to make it happen.

Does a bird sit around worrying & stressing itself out all day trying to fly?

No. It just flies! A bird doesn't even have to think about it because it is innate within the birds DNA.

In the same way self-conception is innate within the DNA of most Female True Beings. Remember only True Beings or Real humans were created by the One True God so only they have this ability to create.

Fake humans or demons were created by the demiurge as shown in all ancient text & in the book of genesis.

On page fifty-three of the brilliant book PARTHENOGENESIS: WOMENS LONG LOST ABILITY TO SELF CONCEIVE by Den Poitras, we learn that an ancient tribe of people called the Ojibwa looked for young girls in the community who had attributes of grace, compassion, intelligence & a love of Truth. When they found such a girl she was instructed in the art of self-conception & kept away from men.

He goes on to quote anthropologist E.S heartland's book; The Supernatural Birth in Relation to The Family. 1909, "The belief in divine birth among indigenous people, worldwide arises not from ignorance of the physiological process of conception, since where it is held, these people claim that there are TWO METHODS of conception. A lower or animal one (through sex.) and a higher one (self-conception.) both are possible & both have occurred." Words in brackets mine.

It is my belief that even if you feel you have had normal pregnancies before your CP if you look
Back on them you will notice that they may have been a CP pregnancy that just turned normal.

Did you feel pregnant for months before your cycle stopped & your tests where positive?

Did you go to the doctor & ask for help & when none was given did you just accept you were not pregnant then months later you suddenly got a positive test?

Did your dates on your first scan not fit the timeline for the dates you had sex?

Or maybe you never had sex at all, yet you have already had a healthy baby. You just didn't tell anyone. You see most CP women who self conceives ONLY conceive in that way.

The higher way.

Women who can't self-conceive, normally conceive in the animal / sexual way.

I can feel the medical cartel chocking on their words as I write this but it's all good. Similar to Jesus, I didn't come to bring peace & unity but a sword, the sword of Truth & one thing demons & programmed sceptical robots HATE, is the Truth.

However, I'll add a sweetener for the medical cartel just because.
Professor Jacques Loeb of Stanford university produced SCIENTIFIC evidence of self-conception in 1912. You can read about his experiments in his book, THE MECHANISTIC CONCEPTION OF LIFE. He came up with the Ovist Theory which states that the foetus can develop from the female ovum alone IF the right amount of electrical charge i.e., Life Force Energy is added to it, & often does not need any male sperm to do so.

So yes, some women can self-conceive & bring the baby to term & I believe that these women often have cryptic pregnancies.

Notice how this confirms very nicely what the indigenous people knew inherently yet science in its great wisdom often called these people savages. How very shameful but they will have the last laugh in the next world.

So, Professor Loeb proved that some women could self-conceive just as I have said but the theory of conception today is epigenesis: the theory of the egg & the sperm.

Yet this theory has never been proven to be the ONLY method of conception it's just the only one that's been promoted.
However, it suited our male dominated society to cover up most of Loeb's work whilst only promoting epigenesis, because the medical cartel can't allow people to understand that there are super women on the planet today who literally do not need a man or even science to have a baby.

I would challenge any scientist to please email me via my Facebook page NEO BROWN evidence of epigenesis being the ONLY method of human conception. I shall be waiting with bated breath.

Here's another important piece of evidence.

In July 1956, a woman in Britain called Emmimarie Jones claimed that her eleven-year-old daughter Monica was unfathered & conceived without a man.

According to the Manchester Guardian, "to prove her claim she submitted to six months of testing by a research team of eminent British doctors."

Their verdict? The newspaper continued, "we have been unable to prove that any man took part in the creation of this child. All our results are consistent with a case of virgin birth. We found nothing in the child that could have come from anyone but the mother."

Now I can hear you thinking, but they didn't have proper DNA testing back then.

True, yet you will see from the case study of Alice in chapter six that after recent DNA testing, both of her CP children have interesting, unusual DNA that proved parthenogenesis had occurred.

Now you know why the branding for this book the female X chromosome is.

The fact is that CP babies who were self-conceived ONLY have the mothers DNA as these doctors proved back in 1956. The child can be male or female of course.
Bottom line: when your friends & family say you don't really need that disrespectful man in your life, they are 100% correct if you are a True Being female going through a CP because you probably self-conceived that child.

You didn't even need that man to get pregnant so why are you putting up with his mess? & No, you do not need to keep him around because you think he's the father of the baby specially not if he is abusive. Kids don't need that kind of father in their lives. I don't care how much you love him.

Now is the time to break free.

In chapter six we will examine the case study of CP mother Sophia from New York who had the courage to leave her unhealthy relationship because she understood she had self-conceived her baby, so he wasn't the father. She then reconnected with her first love; the CP pregnancy turned normal & now they are one happy family.

5.
How to be pregnant with a CP & live & look like you're not

If you've been feeling pregnant with negative tests for more than four months chances, are you are beginning to grow a belly. This is normal because you are really pregnant (see chapter one for how to prove this to yourself.) BUT & this is probably one of the most important things you will ever read: During a CP You do not have the luxury to be able to look or act pregnant until you are confirmed by a doctor!

I know it's beyond hard. I know it's unfair. I know you just want to curl up, cry & hide.
I know you're angry. I know you want to convince your partner, your doctor, your best friend & your family that you really are pregnant but just please remember that we are in a war & as Jesus & other avatars have said, in this world if you are an important True Being, you will have trouble.

This planet is not our turf so the sufferings of life including a CP are of course from the evil god Jehovah & his fake humans & demons in the medical cartel who refuse to use common sense to understand that a CP woman is actually pregnant by checking for a fetal heartbeat.

This is the reason your suffering continues because if they had a shred of real intelligence not to mention integrity, any medical professional would use a doppler & a finger pulse to confirm pregnancy in the face of valid pregnancy symptoms & negative pregnancy tests.

I watched a real-life story of a CP woman on the show I didn't know I was pregnant (most of these women were having a CP it's just they were lucky enough to suddenly gave birth. Why? This will be covered in chapter seven.) who's chiropractor diagnosed her pregnancy by just using a fetal   doppler & found the baby's heartbeat. The woman had gone to the chiropractor with extreme abdominal pain. Once they both realised, she was not only pregnant but in full labour she was rushed to hospital & her baby was born perfectly healthy a few hours later.

I have seen CP women in some of the CP online groups proudly show off their large CP belly & when they don't deliver at forty weeks, they still walk around with no shame looking pregnant & not even trying to hide it.

You may think I'm being harsh, but I have BEEN there. I let myself get all big & pregnant looking with one of my CP babies but thankfully had the common sense to lose weight before people started asking questions.

A very dear CP friend of mine Hannah from the UK explained to me how she too was led by God every step of the way during her three-year CP. "l looked nine months pregnant when I was nine months pregnant, but I trusted God. I just knew that somehow everything would be all right. My tests where still negative when they threw me a baby shower at work, but I kept the faith.

By the time I was almost ten months pregnant people were starting to look at me funny at work & ask questions. But something on the inside just told me to say when they asked about the baby that I didn't want to talk about it. It really was that simple, so people stopped asking about the baby. What you told me about eating like a bird really helped me too because as I changed my diet, ate less & wore baggy clothes to hide my shrinking bump I felt much better about everything. I still knew I was pregnant & my tests were still negative, but not looking pregnant anymore helped me to cope & live my life until about a year later my pregnancy tests turned positive & my cycle finally stopped."

Hannah went on to have a beautiful healthy baby boy, an immense joy to her as she already had three daughters. We shall pick up Hannah's story in chapter six.

Once you realise that you are in a spiritual war you will do anything you can with Gods help to protect yourself & your CP baby.

1. Please do not try to convince your partner, family, or friends that you are really pregnant as they won't believe you.

How can they? They are not in your body, they don't feel the baby moving as you do so because your tests are negative & you have probably taken them to at least one doctor's appointment with you, they just haven't got the ability to comprehend it. Don't blame them just STOP talking about it.

As Mary did during her pregnancy with Jesus, she kept those things in her heart & just spoke to God about it. He kept her going & he will keep you going too.

You are welcome to join my secrete Facebook group the cryptic pregnancy files. I can read peoples energy very well even just from a photo so only sincere women are in my CP group.

If you are married or with a man who is a good man & you are happy with him this is even more reason NOT to try to convince him, you are pregnant UNTIL your pregnancy tests are all big fat positives because you don't want to lose him & you honestly could if you keep insisting the doctors are wrong & you are right!

No man wants to be with a crazy woman & trust me, everyone in the medical cartel will try & convince him you are just that if you keep insisting you are pregnant.

Remember the medical cartel MADE UP something they call a phantom or delusional pregnancy to HIDE the Truth about a CP. Just as they say most people with expanded awareness & who have supernatural experiences are mentally ill.

You could also risk being labelled mentally ill by those blind doctors & put into hospital & pumped full of poisonous drugs. I have heard about this happening to CP women who continued to insist to the medical cartel they were pregnant. This is very frightening but remember there is a WAR on CP Truth so be diligent. Be as wise as serpents & as gentle as doves so always remain calm when dealing with so called medical professionals. Ask God for wisdom & strength at these times.

Honestly, until your tests turn positive it's best to stay away from them unless of course you have any kind of medical emergency.

2. Try & stay slim during a CP

Patrica Cloyd Carter authored a book in 1957 called Come Gently Sweet Lucina that really turned some heads in the pregnancy & childbirth community as she, amongst other things promoted the idea that women should do all they can to keep slim during pregnancy. She ate like a bird, walked a lot, avoided all sugar & even wore high heels right up until the birth of her babies, so she had to be quite slim to manage walking in heels when she was full term! To prove it, on page twenty-eight below is a picture of Patrica just five minutes before the home birth of her ninth child. She looked amazingly relaxed & only around six months pregnant if that & of course the baby was born perfectly healthy & very easily. She attributed her quick & easily births partly to the fact that she had been careful to not put on a lot of weight during her pregnancies.

This unhealthy idea of being able to eat exactly what you want when you want during pregnancy is dangerous for so many reasons & much more so if you are having a cryptic pregnancy.

The medical cartel often try & tell pregnant women who have let themselves put on a lot of weight that they will burn it off quickly after the birth through breast feeding, but trust me, I have been there & this is just not true. Pregnant or CP women who are obese have a much higher risk of developing serious pregnancy & birth related complications, plus their babies are extremely hard to see on ultrasound.

I can't stress how important it is for your emotional & mental health to stay as slim as you can during a CP because if you look pregnant whilst your tests are negative you could have a complete emotional breakdown specially as some CP's last for years.

If you are smart enough to stay slim whilst you might feel pregnant, life is so much easier with a CP if you do not look pregnant.

Let's assume you've let yourself look pregnant & you have a baby bump as I did with one of my CPs, but your pregnancy tests are still negative.

You can lose weight without hurting the baby as babies take what they need first from what you eat so as long as you are not dieting to the extent you feel dizzy & weak, you're good.

Eat when you are hungry & don't deny yourself food obviously but only eat healthy things in small portions. Eat like a bird.

You need a lot of protein during a CP & any pregnancy so milk, eggs, cheese, beans & meat.

This is not the best time to be vegan but be led by your own intuition on what's right for you as with everything.
I repeat my motto for this book & anything I say is believe what you like as ether way I'm good.
Let your OWN intuition guide you on anything I or anyone else has to say about your CP including your doctor.

I know CP women who have lost their CP baby because they listened to their doctor & not their gut so, please don't be one of them.

Drink plenty of water specially in hot weather, avoid sodas or switch to diet soda & avoid all sugary foods, cakes, sweet & junk food. A good rule is if you like salty snacks like soup, cheese, olives, eggs & salads, or crackers it will be a lot easier to remain slim.

Don't ever think, I can eat that extra desert because I'm pregnant. Women having a normal pregnancy often think like this & as a result have over two stone to shift once the baby is born.

Again, I know as I am speaking from experience.

If you find you are constantly hungry due to your CP, you could try diet pills. This might be controversial but so is believing you are pregnant if your tests are negative right?
Some caffeine based over the counter appetite suppressant pills work well but the best thing is to do your own research around this subject & do what's best for you. Simple things like chewing gum or having a diet soda can help if you find you are constantly hungry.

Avoid high impact exercise like the gym or running for obvious reasons. Walking to me is the best exercise & I lost a lot of weight during my CP just by walking for forty minutes four or five times a week.

If you eat like I've described & do the walking, remember to build up to about forty minutes if you are not used to walking for extended periods of time, you could lose six to eight pounds in just a few months if you stick to it. I know I did.

Wear baggier clothes whether you look pregnant or not as you will obviously go up a few bra sizes if you are CP & there's not much you can do about that.
Buy clothes in bigger sizes & don't be tempted into buying any maternity clothes until your CP turns normal as it's just far too depressing.

Once you are looking less pregnant, & as long as you are feeling the baby move regularity, don't worry because you are still pregnant even if you no longer look it.

You can then try & live your life normally as much as possible until your CP turns normal & trust me, you will thank me for that.

Carrying around a big pregnant belly constantly reminds you that you are pregnant with negative tests & the trick is to NOT remind yourself!

You need to focus on the good things in your life & FORGET about your CP to a certain extent.

Many CP women myself included with one of my CP babies felt pregnant, tests were negative & the cycle continued so we forgot about it & carried on with life & after a time the cycle suddenly stopped & bang big fat positive pregnancy test! This often happens with CP women under thirty-five but if you are older you have to be more aware of your CP to some extent as you could have health complications. I will cover this in THE DANGERS OF IGNORING A CP in chapter eight.

3. How to cope emotionally whilst having a CP

This is a big one. How do you avoid extreme sadness & depression whilst going through a CP?

How do you get out of bed every day? How do you go to work, take care of your family & continue in your relationships when you know you're pregnant but because your tests are negative the medical cartel refuse you prenatal care & nobody believes you?

Will you ever smile again? How can you be relaxed & happy?

As Buddha said the more you detach from a situation the better off you are. This is a Gnostic & metaphysics book first so I will always bring everything back to Gnostic Truths because these Truths set me free from a CP. When hellish situations like a CP happen you must not allow your emotions to be drained by it & may your God or your gods help you with this as that's the key.

Don't mourn the loss of a baby. You haven't had a miscarriage & you haven't lost a child.

Ok, you can't be as happy about your CP as a woman with a confirmed pregnancy, but you are halfway there. You are more pregnant than someone who isn't. You must just work on making your baby WANT to show itself. Studies have been done on how babies in the womb can feel your extreme stress or sorrow & sadness & this in turn PROLONGS a CP.

I know it's a vicious circle because you are extremely stressed due to the CP but ironically letting go of the sadness, frustration & stress will help to turn your CP normal. You at least have hope & hope is precious. Practically speaking you must do a pregnancy text at least once a week even if your cycle continues. Why? Well, a lot of women with normal confirmed pregnancies continue to have a cycle, the cycle isn't really the important thing. (See chapter three.) The only important thing is whether your pregnancy tests are positive or not & yes, you can have positive pregnancy tests & still continue to have a cycle.

Buying pregnancy test strips in bulk is the cheapest way to test. If you do get a positive, try other brand tests. Yes, this can be expensive but once your pregnancy tests start turning positive you will want to check with varied brands because the last thing you want is to have a positive at home & a negative at the doctor's office. Doctors almost always use non sensitive pregnancy tests so you will have to have clear big fat positives on at least three different brands of pregnancy tests before you go to the doctor for confirmation.

When I had my first child over twenty years ago there were only a few pregnancy tests on the market & only ever one test in the box.

These days the average pregnancy test has at least two or three tests in the box & it seems there are hundreds of different type of pregnancy tests, most of them early.

Now it has been said & shown scientifically that later in pregnancy you produce several types of HCG. This might be partly why it's so hard for CP women to get positive tests as most pregnancy tests these days only detect the very early form of HCG, because I'm telling you there were no early

pregnancy tests twenty years ago. You waited until you were a week late & took ONE pregnancy test, if it was positive showed it to your doctor, he said congratulations you are pregnant, then he booked you in for your first scan which was almost always at the four-month mark.

Now it's a whole different ball game. Even women with normal pregnancies are paranoid & feel they need two hundred positive pregnancy tests before they can go to the doctor for confirmation. Something is very wrong with this picture.

But I digress.

Remember, when you are testing keep this from your partner because he will think you are nuts. Ok, ok, if you want to be all Romeo & Juliette about it, tell him & don't keep secrets but at least you have been warned.

Do not go out & buy baby supplies until your tests are positive AND you've been confirmed by a doctor as this is just beyond depressing for obvious reasons.

As much as you can, you should switch off from your CP & do not let it dominate your thoughts so you can live your life. Again, this will be so much easier if you do not allow yourself to LOOK pregnant but do not shut your mind off from it to the extent that you don't want to test. That's going from one extreme to the other & ignoring it as I have said, can be very dangerous as you will see in chapter eight.

So, try & strike a happy medium, don't forget about your CP, make sure to test but don't get obsessed with it.

Keep as busy as you can as the quote, "An idle mind is the devil's playground," couldn't be more true concerning a CP as the more time you have to think the more you will be tempted to dwell on things & upset yourself. You can get through this, I did & many have so start a new hobby, begin a new course, or go through that box set you promised yourself.

I remember when I just gave up on my CP sat down & and watched the whole XFLIES box set. I'm so glad I did because it changed my life.

There is a wider reality out there, but most can't or won't see it. That's why I named this book The Cryptic Pregnancy Files because again, many won't understand this book & will condemn it, but they are just useless programmed sceptics & robots. I didn't create this book for the wider public but for the few gifted True Beings who have the eyes to see & the ears to hear REAL CP TRUTH & the ability to put those Truths into practice so they can be free of a CP by turning it into a normal pregnancy & go on to have a healthy CP baby.

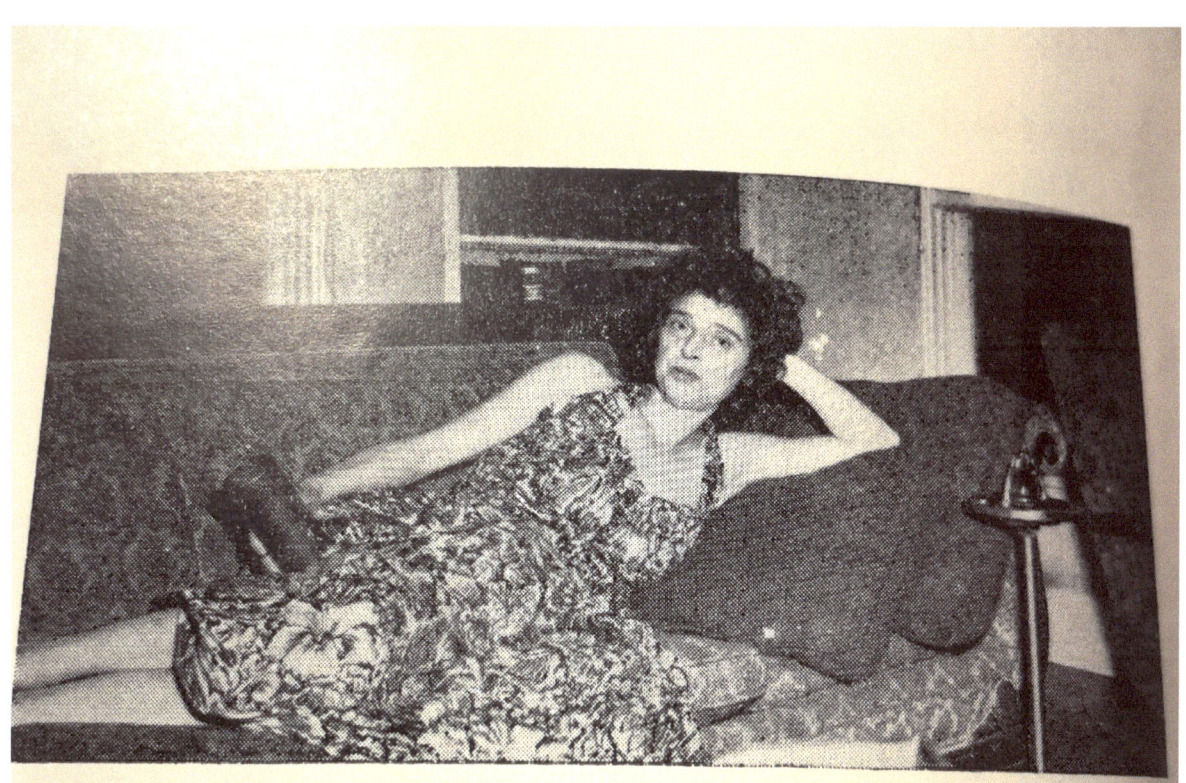

PHOTO BY MARY LOU CULBERTSON, REPORTER "DAYTONA NEWS JOURNAL"

SERENE WAITING

Five minutes before Mrs. Carter's ninth child was born.

6.

Case studies of women who had healthy CP babies

This will be a very positive chapter for those of you who are currently going through a CP.

The women in these case studies are women I ether know personally or whose stories have been verified. Many sent me doctors & scan reports. Names have been changed of course to maintain their privacy.

But you're not a doctor you say. This is correct but most people should be able to read & understand medical reports. If not, why are patients & family ever offered them?

Exactly.

We met Hannah in chapter five so let's continue with her CP story.

Hannah had split up with her partner by the time she was past her due date. She then lost a lot of weight following the advice I give about diet & exercise during a CP.

She no longer looked pregnant & got on with life still knowing that she WAS pregnant.

She had a strong faith in God & was an obvious True Being. Her intuition was razor sharp regarding her own CP & knew before I did that most CP babies are self-conceived.

When she had been CP for around two years she got back with her ex-partner & she was ecstatic.

Not LOOKING pregnant she was of course able to sleep with him as normal. Another big reason to keep slim during a CP is your partner. Whilst some guys like larger ladies, if you continue to have a big pregnant belly after nine months the situation will come between you in more ways than one.

Hannah had been back with her partner Dan for a few months when she missed her cycle. She took a pregnancy test & it was positive!

I remember she called me sounding so excited & before I could congratulate her, she said, "Neo I know it's the same baby. Although I had lost belly & most of the CP weight around ten months CP, I STILL felt the baby move every day. I've been pregnant four times now & have three daughters; I know what baby movement feels like!" I didn't doubt it. "I don't know how but I just think because I've been so happy & full of hope & joy for a change since I've been back together with Dan, it somehow tuned my tests positive. I can't explain it, but this is what my intuition & my spirit are telling me."

I didn't think about it much at the time because I was worried about her going to the doctor with her positive test because after going to them for help during her CP & being almost laughed at for daring

to disagree with the great white coats, I wondered how they would take the news of this confirmed pregnancy. Would they make her do a billion pregnancy tests just to be sure? Or was her positive test just a one off?

This can happen during a CP sadly.

Your cycle can stop, you can have a few nice positives but then your cycle starts up again & your tests are negative. It's heart-breaking & also why some women think they have a miscarriage every other month or so. Most women are not having an early miscarriage at all they are just pregnant with a CP baby & it would be great if they knew this as then at least they wouldn't have to mourn the loss of a baby that they really didn't lose at all.

The reason a CP can turn normal & go back to CP again will be covered in the next chapter. Everything is about Energy on this planet so the cure to a CP is metaphysical yet at the same time very practical.

A few months later she called with the good news, "so I waited three months before going to the doctor. My cycle didn't return & I didn't do any more pregnancy tests, but I just knew they would stay positive."

Again, I was amazed at Hannah's great faith & strength. I knew most women would have been ether testing every day to make sure the tests stayed positive or running to the doctor as soon as they had the first big fat positive, but not Hannah. She was a True CP warrior.

So went on, "I wanted to kind of trick the doctors as they had been so rude & unhelpful to me when my tests were negative. I also wanted to see what they would say because I know I can feel the same kind of fetal movement that I've felt since I was five months CP so how far along would they say I am seeing as I've just had a positive test, yet I know I've been pregnant with a CP for two years already? So, I went to A&E but didn't tell them about missing my cycle or having a positive pregnancy test, I just told them I'd been feeling sick & very run down so they ran a pregnancy test just to be safe."

I'll never forget how I laughed out loud when she said, "The doctors came back in the room & said you're pregnant & I acted all surprised! They then ran a pregnancy blood test & according to that test I was only SIX WEEKS PREGNANT!" I knew instinctively that this was definitely not the case as she had been feeling movement & had of course used my Finger Pulse & Doppler Test for confirmation when she was around five months CP.

You just can't feel a six-week foetus move & she had been feeling a lot of movement that day as she did most days during her CP, "I didn't say anything Neo I just went along with it. I mean what's the point of disagreeing with a doctor. You never get anywhere. I was just really grateful I was finally confirmed. I didn't have a scan until I was five months pregnant by their calculation, but I knew I was really two & a half years pregnant with my CP baby by then. Sure enough, when I went for the scan, they said the baby was measuring right along with being five months gestation."

As these babies are often self-conceived it's not such a stretch of the imagination to understand that they may grow differently & may produce lower amounts of HCG than babies who were not self-conceived.

Happily, Hannah went on to be induced & have a beautiful healthy baby boy, the son she had always longed for when she was thirty-nine weeks pregnant by the doctor's calculations, but almost three years CP by her own.

After at least three years studying & researching a CP this was the first positive CP story I heard & I was very grateful for it.

Obviously, sceptics will laugh at such a story & say Hannah was definitely not pregnant for three years & when she got her positive pregnancy test it was a brand-new pregnancy.

But CP Truths are for those who have the Nous or knowing within them. Although very few people do these days, the CP Truth in this book will resonate with them & help them greatly.

Bottom line: the Truth is always exclusive not inclusive.

Sophia was a very cool twenty something from New York who joined my old yahoo CP group already understanding a lot about her CP. Her partner at the time ALSO believed in & accepted her CP. This was rare.

Unfortunately, the relationship wasn't a good one as he was very controlling.

Thankfully, she found the strength to leave him quite early in her CP & actually told me she felt that God would bring her the right man & father for her CP baby because she knew she had self-conceived the baby so had no guilt about meeting someone new.

This is key. Truth is if you have self-conceived your baby you will know about it because you will be shown this. If you are not shown or led to this Truth yourself & you are happy with your partner just keep quite & keep slim & the baby will show itself when you understand & follow the advice in chapter seven.

CP babies who have been self-conceived ONLY have the mothers DNA. Find this hard to believe? Then Let's leave Sophia's story for a moment & meet Alice.

Alice already had two children. She knew there was something very special about them as they were both extremely gifted, (CP baby's often grow to be very gifted children & adults.) So, she took them to the doctor who wanted to run some intelligence tests & some blood tests.

I'll let Alice tell her story, "When I went to the doctor for the children's results, she seemed quite nervous. She showed me the blood lab results & I realised they had also run DNA tests which I thought strange. The doctor said she had never seen DNA test results like this in all her twenty plus years of practice because my children's DNA, contained no MALE or PATERNAL DNA at all.

"The doctor said it meant that all of each of my children's DNA ONLY contained MATERNAL DNA. She really wanted to run more tests on my kids, but I got a bad feeling about it because I felt the
Doctors might treat them like lab rats or something. I made a polite excuse & left with the DNA results."

I have personally seen these result & yes both of her children a girl & a boy had 100% of their mother's maternal DNA.

I'll give you a second to let that sink in.

These results proved to me that Alice had self-conceived her children plus Alice was actually going through a CP at the time so as it progressed, we spoke & figured out that her two children had probably been CP pregnancies also.

Why? Well, because she had felt off, sick & pregnant a good few months, maybe six or seven she said, before she got a positive with both children. During this time, her cycle continued but was lighter.

She was young at the time so didn't stress about it.

When she looked back on her pregnancies in the light of her current CP & the information, I had given her about self-conception, she was able to join the dots herself & realise that for her at least, cryptic pregnancies are often selfconceived. Of course, the fact that both children had a 100% of her DNA & zero paternal DNA confirmed this.

Going back to Sophia, when she was around twelve months CP, & a few months after her split she reconnected with her high school sweetheart.

They were an extremely happy couple & yes you guessed it, soon her cycle stopped & her pregnancy tests turned positive. Like Hannah Sophia knew the   pregnancy was the same CP pregnancy she had been having all along & felt really relieved the baby didn't show up in her previous relationship.
She felt no guilt about hiding her CP from her new boyfriend until it turned positive as why should she have any guilt? She knew she had self-conceived the baby plus if you can't convince a medical doctor you're pregnant with negative tests when all the doctor has to do is use common sense & a finger pulse to find your heartbeat & a doppler, to find the baby's once you are at last five months CP, then how can you convince anyone? You can't & you shouldn't try to as I've pointed out in previous chapters.

Sophia's pregnancy was of course confirmed & she went on to have a beautiful healthy baby girl by c section.

Again, only those who are very awake spiritually or to use the Gnostic term real humans & True Beings can accept these things. To most this will appear to be untenable but as always, my motto is:
 believe what you like as ether way I'm good. It makes no difference to me in the slightest what you think or believe about me & my work because I'm obviously not revealing these kinds of Truths to be popular.

Carla wasn't particularly spiritual or awake sadly. She worked as a nurse & almost worshiped the medical profession. She would never question or second guess a doctor, but she did read medical articles about women suddenly going into labour & was smart enough to understand the obvious Truth that:

Most of these women HAD been going through a CP but as their pregnancy tests were negative & their cycle continued, they didn't question it.

Carla wasn't going to let it go & be convinced that once she went into labour at nine months, she would tell the doctors exactly what she'd been going through for months as she had really been pregnant, but her tests had just been negative.

She had an older child so knew what fetal movement felt like. She also used my Finger Pulse & Doppler Test & found a second heartbeat of 140bpm in her belly whilst hers on a finger pulse at the same time was only 65bpm.

Her belly was growing normally & by six months CP she looked six months pregnant so she paid for a private scan, having felt a lot of movement from five months CP & having had a normal pregnancy & delivery before, Carla was convinced they would find the baby.

Except of course the private scan didn't find the baby.

The only thing they found was an empty uterus. Carla was devastated because she wasn't going to doubt medical technology or the science as she believed she was far too smart for that.

However, if she really were pregnant with negative tests how could her uterus be empty?

Let me tell you what happened to me during a CP pregnancy. I had a lot of pain when I would have been around seven months CP & went to hospital for a scan.
As the doctor did the scan & I looked at the grey screen I saw as plain as day, for maybe five seconds a baby's skull turned towards me as if it were looking right at me, with its tiny white teeth in its gums just as I had seen my son in his scan during my previous normal pregnancy when he was around seven months gestation.

"Look! Can't you see it?" I told the doctor.

The doctor said there was nothing there at all.

Obviously, I had told the doctors I had been feeling pregnant when I went in & as I had a bit of a belly, they ran a pregnancy test but of course it was negative.

Now as this has happened to me, I know from my own experience that for whatever reasons if your pregnancy test is negative doctors are NOT allowed to tell you there is a baby on the scan.
End of story.

Sometimes it's for a simple reason like a doctor can't bill you for pregnancy if your tests are negative.
Sometimes they have to lie because this is what their higher ups tell them to do when finding a woman pregnant with a CP.

The illuminati / elite whatever your pet name for the extremely wealthy people who run the planet, DO NOT want the world to knew that some women can not only be pregnant with negative tests, but can carry for years & more importantly, many have actually self-conceived their CP baby & this can even be proved by doing a simple DNA test once it's born because like Alice's children, it would almost certainly have maternal DNA only.
A Mexican CP lady, Elena who I knew from my CP group called me one day sounding very scared as she literally had men in black go in & threaten her doctor she feels, as she waited in the waiting room for her appointment. Elena had convinced her doctor on the phone to try The Finger Pulse & Doppler Test at her next appointment, but the doctor

point blank refused when she went in & kept telling her very loudly that she was definitely not pregnant & she needed to drop it.

Why did that doctor who had seemed so cooperative on the phone the day before suddenly change her mind after the visitors dressed in black & who exactly where they?

The illumiNUTS (illuminati) do what they have always done to try & hide the Truth: they ridicule those who know about the subject they want to hide because nobody wants to be ridiculed so said person will often give up.

Except for me perhaps because I just don't care.

So, Carla's scan showing an empty uterus is really no surprise.

However, Carla accepted it & dropped her CP knowledge & my group like a hot brick, lost loads of weight & then, less than a year later, was telling anyone who would listen on her FB page that she was finally really pregnant & happily posted pictures of her many clear positive pregnancy tests.

Of course, in light of what we have just seen it was probably the same CP baby all along.

Carla was only twenty-four so forgetting about her CP & losing a lot of weight quickly didn't harm her or the baby as she went on to have a healthy pregnancy & baby, but was induced as most women are, at around thirty-nine weeks. I know she definitely had the baby, although she was no longer in my CP group, because she began making YouTube videos about her pregnancy & the baby as soon as it was born.

The saddest CP story I ever heard was a CP woman I saw on YouTube telling her story years ago.

She said she had been pregnant for five years.

She had two big folders full of her medical notes beside her & had a big pregnant belly. She looked full term to me. I don't remember her name, but I do remember her describing her last scan
 appointment, "My doctor finally gave me another scan & he asked me how long I thought I'd been pregnant. I was four years at the time, so I told him. As he looked at the scan his eyes grew wide & he said, 'This is impossible! You can't still be pregnant at four years!' Yet I could see what he could see: a full-term baby on that scan as plain as day. This doctor actually started to shake. He said I couldn't be pregnant at all as he knew my pregnancy tests were negative, he said I should be dead by now & he couldn't believe what he was seeing. He told me to please leave his office & to never come back. That's when I stopped going to doctors for help."

Back then I'd never known a CP woman to go over three years but sadly many do. She looked resigned yet strangely peaceful.

I'll never forgot the last thing she said on that video. "I believe in Jesus & the bible says there is a friend who sticks closer than a brother & he ain't lying, he ain't lying."

I felt heartbroken for her. I wanted to cry but more than that I was angry. Angry at the injustice of a CP & the hell the medical cartel put CP women through.
 It is with this Energy of righteous indignation that I use to author this book to expose Real CP Truth so that CP women all over the world will finally have the ability to fix their cryptic pregnancies & holding their heads up high, feel not shame but pride in front of the feeble-minded medical cartel when they finally get their confirmation by using the information in this book.

7.
How to fix a CP

> Everything is energy & that's all there is too it.
>
> Albert Einstein

First of all, do you release that there is ZERO evidence to prove that pregnancy only lasts for nine months or forty weeks to be exact?

Historically there have been three main theories or ideas about why a woman goes into labour at nine months: The mother producing oxytocin, the feel-good love hormone, the baby's lungs being fully developed so that they signal for labour to begin, or some think the baby's adrenal glands might be the signal that starts labour.

But these ideas are only THEORIES.

What is a theory?

A theory is just an idea.
So, wait a minute, CP women worldwide are laughed at ridiculed, ignored & called crazy by the medical cartel JUST because our EXPERIENCE not our IDEA, of pregnancy is different from the traditional IDEA of pregnancy length?

You have to be kidding right?

No sadly I'm not.

Now, even if we take these three main ideas which are not PROVEN facts there are many questions that need to be asked.

How much oxytocin does a woman need to produce to start her labour for example? Supposing she stops producing it? Does it mean labour always stops? If so for how long? What concentration does the hormone have to be in the blood & is the amount different for each pregnant woman, or is it a one size fits all amount?

The same kinds of questions can be asked for the other two theories. The medical cartel has no answers for these simple questions, however.

Funny that.

I don't care what your idea or religious medical doctrines are doc, I only care about the TRUTH & since I know many CP women who have been & are pregnant for much longer than nine months, your nine-month pregnancy idea as tradition is plain idiotic, SPECIALLY as even if a woman with a confirmed pregnancy starts labour at nine months she almost ALWAYS stops!

This is why over 90% of women are induced when their labour starts & STOPS at nine months. From the braking of the waters to induction drugs, to manual dilation of the cervix to a c section, only an extremely small percentage of women who begin their labour at thirty-eight to forty weeks have the baby quickly & easily in hospital or with a midwife without any medical interventions at all.

Supposing these women began labour then when it stopped, they were sent home?

Would they just give birth at home as there is no stopping labour once it starts?

Of course, this is exactly what the medical cartel would have you believe but you will NEVER know for sure as the only pregnant women who are sent home when their labour begins at nine months are women with cryptic pregnancies.

Women with confirmed pregnancies are not allowed out of the hospital until that baby is born & like I said, almost all labouring women in a hospital or with a midwife have SOME form of medical intervention to get that baby out. So how can pregnancy be nine months?

In 2012 a new idea about why labour begins at nine months in humans & can't possibly go on for longer (despite the fact that, as I have said over 90% of women are induced once labour starts & stops because it always stops.) is the idea that the mother's metabolism, not the size of her birth canal as some previously thought, is the real reason that human gestation is only nine months.
Coined by professor Dunsworth of the University of Rhode Island, the theory suggests that the reason women do not carry past nine months is because she cannot support the baby & herself metabolically as humans can only use so many calories a day.

I beg to differ.

Long distance runners use many more calories a day than say an office worker.

We have all met women who are very slim yet seem to eat a lot. How many calories a day would they burn in pregnancy? probably much more than the woman who doesn't seem to eat much yet finds it's hard to lose weight.

If Dunsworths metabolic idea of human gestation is correct then women who burn more calories a day, because they have a naturally high metabolic rate, should have shorter gestations then women whose bodies do not burn calories as quickly.

So logically there should be a HUGE VARIATION in human gestation.

But of course, these very simple logical questions are never answered by Dunsworth because the great white coat has spoken & just like the Spanish Inquisition, we mere mortals are not allowed to question the myths & doctrines of the mainstream religion of our day, which of course is medicine & science.

Even if Dunsworths idea holds water, not all human women on earth have the same type of DNA therefore there simply cannot be a one size fits all for metabolic rate during pregnancy & therefore gestation length.

There have been cases of people who have a three even four strand DNA. We have already shown that some women can self-conceive so it would be logical to conclude that their DNA & biology must be different from women who can't conceive in this way.

I would have thought that would be quite obvious & no, I'm not saying some women are elite compared to others because they possess the ability to self-conceive, they are just different.

Is a bird better than a cat because it can fly whilst the cat can only dart up a tree?

No. The cat & the bird are just different.

If this is the case & it is, would it be so hard to understand that because of biological differences, proven by the fact that some women can & do self-conceive, the fact that these women's biology ALSO enables them to have much longer gestations or keep a pregnancy hidden for years shouldn't be so hard to understand. Of course, NOBODY wants to be pregnant for years but that doesn't mean it DOESN'T happen.

Unless of course you are extremely faithful to the religious traditions of the medical cartel & refuse to think for yourself like most programmed sceptics.
The saddest thing is, it is purely because they are so programmed that they can't see.
Like a broken tv from the 80s with only one channel.

As a True Being created by the Great Spirit/ The Absolute every situation & every social interaction will ether drain your Life Force & pollute you or add to your Life Force & enhanced it.

To turn a cryptic or a hidden pregnancy into a normal pregnancy i.e.: your cycle stops & your pregnancy tests are positive, takes a huge amount of Life Force or chi.

To suddenly, almost painlessly and very quickly, give birth to a CP baby without ever having the pregnancy turn normal (like on the real life show I didn't know I was pregnant.) takes an almost superhuman amount of Life Force. This will be covered in The Cryptic Pregnancy Files volume two.

A True Being or Real human has a particular amount of divine Energy within its soul at birth, but things are rigged in this dimension by the demiurge (Satan / Jehovah.) because in order to keep this world running in energy terms, (I'm talking about spiritual energy not solar energy or fossil fuel.)
The mock beings, fake humans & demons have to do the work of their father the demiurge & drain you of your Life force.

How is your life force drained & polluted?

Causing suffering & emotional trauma are the Two Big devices of spiritual energy drainage on this planet.

Ever met a person who just has bad luck, family trouble & heartache after heartache in life?

Maybe that's you.

That person is probably a True Being.

If your life has always been easy & things just seem to fall into place for you then you probably have no divine Energy or Life Force worth draining so the demiurge doesn't bother with you.

Notice the bible & many religions & a lot of so-called preachers will tell you that tests, trials & suffering come from God to teach you a spiritual lesson.

These are pure illogical LIES.

You do not cause a person untold stress & emotional pain in order to teach them something you just teach them!

But many good people, go to church because they feel the pull of the divine from within them & want to connect with the Truth that's already inside of them. (Remember Jesus did say that the kingdom of God is within you but Newsflash: he wasn't talking to everyone. He was only talking to True Beings as they are the only ones with The Light within.)
Religion & churches drain most True Beings horribly. These systems were created by the demiurge & are run by his demons & fake humans in order to trap the True Being & drain its energy as demons & fake humans LIVE on the spiritual energy they steal from True beings.

This Energy drainage doesn't only happen in religion but in institutions such as your school, college, university, work environment, Hospitals of course, your family relationships & even social interactions.

The obvious things like smoking, drinking, doing drugs & being promiscuous are very bad for your Life Force so please avoid them as much as possible if you are a True Being & you know deep down who you are.

Ok so you can understand that a CP might need a lot of life force to turn it into a normal pregnancy but how exactly can we do this?

I will show you.

The energy loss a CP woman experiences during a CP is catastrophic. Why?

Because of the sheer EMOTIONAL STRESS of the situation.

It's a vicious cycle that starts with her feeling pregnant yet having very faint or negative tests, her cycle stopping or changing to her actually feeling the baby move & kick yet getting zero help from anyone in the medical cartel.

So, she tries to believe the doctors when they tell her she's not pregnant & the movement is just gas & forgets about the pregnancy thing.

But her belly feels hard & round despite the fact that she really watches what she eats.
She has often been through pregnancy before, is already a mother & this feels exactly the same.

In her free time, she tries to research her situation online, she reads other CP women's stories, but nobody has any answers.

Most give in & forget about being pregnant but not in a good way. They just haven't got the spiritual strength or ability to keep themselves awake to the Truth & who can blame them?

Some like Carla in the previous chapter, worship the medical cartel so a no, from them is never questioned logically even in one's own mind sadly.

Ignorance is NOT bliss when it comes to a CP.

CP babies will literally STOP growing if you lose too much vital Life Force and will only start growing again once you have stopped accumulating so much negative Energy. Fact.

So, the CP equation is: Feeling pregnant with negative pregnancy tests =Energy Loss.

    Energy Loss =Lack of life force for the CP to become normal.

    Lack of life force for the CP to become normal =Extended gestation & Negative tests.

    This is the cryptic pregnancy vicious circle.

    This is the first & MAJOR reason a CP continues.

Energy Loss also happens when a True Being interacts with a fake human or demon.

Obviously, you can't see this happening, but you can often feel it. For example, we all know someone at work or even in our family who makes everyone feel drained. They upset people, they make unfair demands of people & worse, they seem to enjoy it.

This kind of behaviour is very normal for a fake human. They have no real morals even if they pretend to because they have no real soul within them. They enjoy arguments or emotionally hurting people.

Most of us are smart enough to avoid these kinds of people as much as we can.

Because all humans look similar, it is impossible without the literal spiritual eyes to see, to be able to understand what consciousness is in each human being we interact with.

Only True Beings or Real humans can read the Energy of a person & now that we are in the very last days the spiritual gift of Sight has been given to us.

Practice this by looking at photos of different people or try reading the energy of people on TV or in films, or people you meet in everyday life.

What kind of Energy radiates from them? Is it nurturing? Does it make you feel calm or uneasy?

Normally your first impression, the thing you feel when you first meet someone is correct.

For example, have you ever been on a date & on paper the person is perfect for you? They even have the look you like but when you actually sit down with them something feels off & you can't put your finger on it. This is your higher self or spirit telling you the person is not for you because their ontology, the spiritual matter their consciousness is composed of, is wrong or even dangerous for you.
True Beings should only date or marry other True Beings. Why would you want to be with a fake human or demon? Your life will be hell & I can testify to the truth of that statement as I have dated fake humans & demons & it's not good to say the least.

Moses in the bible actually helped to separate the Light from the Darkness, the True Being human from the demonic consciousness humans so that they wouldn't interbreed as much.

This is what the ancient text really meant when it said keep the race pure.

It was all about keeping the True Beings pure by not marrying non-True Beings or demons.

This information should be very obvious to spiritual people. Race means nothing, it is only the consciousness within this cardboard box that is your body or the vehicle you use for this planet that is truly important.

For a CP woman having sex or even just living with a partner who is of a demonic consciousness, or a fake human is spiritual suicide.

Having sex with a fake human not only pollutes your precious Life Force it drains it & worse, but the sex can also program you by feelings via your emotional body to not see that guy for who he truly is in spiritual terms.

The saying that love is blind couldn't be more true.

I'm sure we have all been there but being in a relationship with a fake human or demon during a CP WILL prolong your CP 100%.

Amelia's case perfectly illustrates this point.

Amelia was a woman in a toxic relationship but had struggled with a CP BEFORE she got into it.

I knew Amelia from Spurgeon's College London when we both read Theology. She had followed my advice by avoiding unnecessary weight gain & was able to get on with her life completely as she was naturally slim so only had a bit of a belly after meals.

Amelia was very much in love with Simon at first & prayed & prayed that her CP would turn normal now that they were a couple so he could be the father for her CP child. Sex with the RIGHT man, & even the Energy from just being around him CAN often turn a CP normal, which when you think about it would make him the father.

But no matter how much she tested; her pregnancy tests remained stubbornly negative & her cycle continued.
She couldn't understand it as she knew Sophia & Hannah from my CP group & felt that like them, finally being with the right guy would turn her CP normal like it did for them.

But Simon wasn't the right guy.

After a few months cracks begin to appear in his personality.

He broke Her beautiful 70s retro table in a mad rage one night & pulled her flat screen tv off the wall on another.

You couldn't make it up. She soon realised he had extreme physiological problems. He had hidden them very well from her for a long time as they had been friends for years before they got together.

He then became physically abusive & she, believing the Christian lie she was brought up with to love your enemy kept forgiving him as she felt if she loved God & she did, this was her duty.

She still tested regularly but when she did of course her tests were negative & of course her cycle continued.

Amelia might have been blind to the facts, but her CP baby obviously wasn't, so he hid himself.

By this time, she had been CP for a long time & had put on a few pounds.

Simon taunted her again & again about the weight gain but what could she do?

Tell him she was REALLY pregnant? No of course not. Not with negative tests.

She just had to swallow her pain & her pride until one day a kind neighbour who knew what was going on with Simon gave her a kitten as her female cat had just birthed a beautiful litter.

Simon, being a demon of course hated the beautiful tabby kitten.

But the kitten became her lifeline.

He followed Amelia everywhere, sat with her & slept with her whenever he could.

Did you ever meet a pet who was so full of love it seemed angelic? This definitely described Amelia's new kitten who she named Timmy.

Somehow, through the love of that tiny grey kitten as it grew & because she started waking up to pure Gnostic Truth by reading a lot of Dr. Joseph Chiappalone's articles on rense.com she was able to find the strength to end things with Simon.

Predictably, he begged & cried & pleaded for her to change her mind promising he would definitely change this time blah blah blah.

But she was stronger than him & she could finally see him for what he really was.
The next year was one of the happiest of her life!

She had her tiny little house back all to herself. She began work in her dream career of journalism & worked from home because she just hatred to be away from Timmy.

She didn't cry one tear for Simon & definitely didn't miss him. How can you miss a devil?

 She didn't date anyone else ether. Amelia was still CP & didn't look pregnant at all but she sensed she was supposed to do this alone & her career was starting to blow up so she could afford to now.

Soon her cycle stopped.

She began taking pregnancy tests again.

It didn't happen right away but within a few months she had her first positive pregnancy test late one night after finishing an article for work.

She held Timmy & cried with relief because she knew deep down that this was the start of the big fat positive for her cryptic pregnancy.

Soon all of her pregnancy tests, even the hard to pass digitals were clearly positive.

She went to a sexual health clinic for confirmation & on my advice on how to handle the medical cartel once a CP turns normal, (see chapter ten.) had her pregnancy finally confirmed by a doctor.

She had been split up from her ex & hadn't had sex in over a year & a half by the time her pregnancy was confirmed so her CP was self our CP finally turns normal.

As we now know, a CP can stay hidden & is prolonged because of Energy Loss.

Being in a relationship with an abusive partner will result in a huge amount of Energy loss for the CP woman & sex with a guy whose consciousness is demonic or evil (see chapter two.) will not only result in Energy or life force loss but in the ACCUMULATION of negative energy from the partner with the negative consciousness.

So, despite Amelia's initial hope that her CP would finally turn normal as she was in a new relationship with a man she loved, it didn't happen at all.

I cannot stress how dangerous it is for you if you are going through a CP to be in a toxic relationship or even just be sleeping with a toxic guy.

You will know deep down in your gut what I mean as some guys seem to be lovely & are definitely not physically abusive, but they are manipulative & hurt you emotionally.

Even guys who play that new emotional game of ghosting are toxic.

Do not give them a second chance because your Energy loss will result in your CP being prolonged & you don't need that.

You don't even need a man to have a CP baby as you probably didn't even need one to conceive it & you don't need one to turn it normal as Amelia's story proves.

I have known Amelia for many years now & she & her CP child are doing great.

Let's look at the CP equation in the light of Amelia's situation:

CP equation part 2:

Stress from an abusive / toxic relationship during a CP = Negative Energy + Energy Loss.

Sex with a toxic partner during a CP = Negative Energy + Energy Loss.

Negative Energy +Energy Loss = Lack of Life Force for the CP to become normal.

Lack of Life Force for the CP to become normal = Extended gestation & negative tests.

This is a Cryptic Pregnancy vicious circle.

This is the second MAJOR reason a CP continues.

That guy who sang the song Don't Worry Be Happy was right because as the bible says, "The joy of the Lord is your strength."

If you truly belong to the Light IT will give you quite joy & happiness whatever your situation.

Remember to communicate with your CP baby in your heart & tell him or her that it's wanted. Don't blame it for the stress a CP creates as it's not the CP baby's fault, it is the fault of the medical cartel alone.

It's when you let go & don't stress over the CP so much, when you don't let it bother you at all but at the same time you are not ignorant to what is really going on with your body during a CP, that your Life Force is strengthened.

All of the CP women I spoke to whose CPs turned normal, including my own had stopped going to doctors looking for answers very early in their CP.

This was a good thing because as you will see in the next chapter, the medical cartel can & do come up with all sorts of excuses for a CP & often due to trickery, convince some gullible CP women to abort their CP baby.

8.
The dangers of ignoring a CP

One of the very real dangerous of ignoring a CP is the risk of high blood pressure.
I had such high blood pressure in my last CP that at one GP appointment he told me to go straight to hospital as he thought I was going to have a stroke.

I remember rolling my eyes internally & thinking, "Doc, even if I go to the hospital they won't TREAT me for my prolonged CP pregnancy, the REAL reason that my blood pressure is so high so why bother?" This is because a doctor's brain seems to shut down when you say you feel pregnant, but your tests are negative & they point blank REFUSE to do any other tests to try & rule out pregnancy.

Did the ancient women need pregnancy urine & blood tests to tell them they were pregnant? Of course not.

Yet western women are told that if the great god of the HCG test is negative no other tests will be performed to rule out pregnancy & if the woman insists, she is still pregnant with negative tests she is delusional.

Do you know how controlling it is to say someone is delusional for not agreeing with you? Specially as the doctors point blank refuse to look for a fetal heartbeat, one of the things that doctors admit in their own literature should be used to RULE OUT a delusional or a false pregnancy.

Preeclampsia is a dangerous condition of pregnancy that causes very high blood pressure, swelling of the hands, feet, face & kidney damage.

The only cure for PE is delivery of the baby so of course, if you have been CP for more than nine months as most CP women are, you could be in real danger if you develop PE.
This is precisely why ignoring a CP & just blindly believing the medical cartel when they tell you, you are NOT pregnant when your gut, the baby kicking & a second heartbeat on a fetal doppler of 120bpm or more whilst yours on a finger pulse is 60 to 90bpm, is beyond dangerous.

I know it's hard, but you have to find the strength to trust your instincts.

I had preeclampsia in my first pregnancy so learned a lot about how to avoid it.

The lifesaving food type during pregnancy is protein & this to a huge extent protects you against PE.

So, fish, eggs, beans, meat, full fat milk & yogurts should be the bulk of your diet.

Avoid too many complex carbs like breads, baked goods, chips, rice, pasta & pizza. Avoid sugar & if you like fizzy drinks switch to diet as every little helps.

Drink plenty of water & take long walks or build up to them.

After much research I did all of this in my second pregnancy & didn't get preeclampsia thankfully.
I didn't even get high blood pressure.

The term cryptic pregnancy was, as far as I remember, originally coined by myself & other pioneering women in the original online CP community back in 2012 to describe a woman who is actually pregnant but has negative pregnancy tests.
Back then a woman who didn't know she was pregnant until she gave birth was rarer than a red unicorn.

However, it suited the medical cartel & ultimately the illuminati to twist the truth of our original meaning for a cryptic pregnancy so that now most people think a cryptic pregnancy means a woman who doesn't know she is pregnant until she gives birth.

But what's cryptic about that? If anything, that should be called a surprise pregnancy.

Hello?

According to new look wiki updated in 2021, "… The term cryptic pregnancy is ALSO used online for a special form of false pregnancy (pseudocyesis,) or delusion of pregnancy, in which a woman who has no medical verification of pregnancy believes that she is pregnant."
So that would be us but unlike the fairy tale myth the medical cartel made up called a false or delusional pregnancy, CP women know they are pregnant not in the absence of ANY medical verification, but ONLY in the absence of a positive pregnancy test.

Now watch this.

According to WEBMD in a FALSE pregnancy, there is no baby seen on a scan, (this can be for many reasons if you are pregnant with negative tests & we shall cover some of them below.)

& There is NO FETAL HEARTBEAT.

It does not say because a quack, I mean doctor doesn't think the woman is pregnant because her pregnancy tests are negative it is a false pregnancy.

 In summery it says: negative pregnancy tests & no baby seen on a scan AND no fetal heartbeat =
A FALSE pregnancy.

It often suits the doctors to do a quick two second scan if a CP woman insist on one, but they will Almost NEVER try & find a fetal heartbeat.

Funny that isn't it?

So, wiki is lying again but just because the people who write for wiki can't think deductively or logically it doesn't mean the rest of us can't.

You know I feel quite sorry for doctors because when the Truth about a CP comes out & CP women all over the world begin to wake up & stand up to the doctors calmly using the simple & logical common sense in this book, many of them will be sued for negligence because MOST of the medical cartel point blank REFUSE to:

Use the Finger Pulse & Doppler Test. (see cheaper one.) Or try to find a fetal heartbeat on a scan, even just by performing an honest abdominal scan with the sound turned up so that the distinctive sound of a fetal heartbeat, a sound like the galloping of horses, can be heard if it is there.

This is blatant medical negligence.

Always remain very calm when dealing with doctors during a CP. Do not get angry or emotional as this enforces the erroneous notion that CP women are not really pregnant, they are just delusional.

Tell your doctor that you are recording your appointment on your phone & record them on your voice app as evidence should you sue.

Then tell them calmly about the Finger Pulse & Doppler Test & ask them to please perform the test on you so that they can really rule out a FALSE pregnancy.

As I have said before & I will say it forever: NO HUMAN BEING ALIVE HAS TWO SEPARATE HEARTBEATS IN ONE BODY.

The medical cartel admits this in their own medical literature as we have seen because they have said there is NO fetal heartbeat in a false pregnancy & clearly to find NO fetal heartbeat the doctor has to actually LOOK for one in the first place.

Come on now.

If you are at least five months CP an honest abdominal scan, with the SOUND TURNED ON will rule out a false pregnancy as of course there will be no fetal heartbeat sound if it is false.

So why is it that the medical cartel seems to thrive on calling a cryptic pregnancy a false pregnancy yet REFUSE to look honestly for a fetal heartbeat if pregnancy tests are negative & the woman feels pregnant?

Because they prefer lies to the Truth & if they admit that most CP women really WERE pregnant all along, most of the doctors will be sued for damages & a new cryptic pregnancy theory, the theory I am uncovering in this book will have to be adopted by the medical cartel.

& We can't have that now, can we?

Why are scans often empty during a CP?

When a CP woman gets an abdominal scan, she thinks her nightmare is finally over & knows that the doctors will see sense once they see the baby on a scan, even if her pregnancy tests are negative.

I remember the huge sense of hope I felt when I had my first CP scan. I was about six months CP at the time.

But like most CP women nothing was seen on my abdominal scan. They couldn't see a baby. They couldn't see much of anything apparently but why couldn't the baby be seen if I had performed the Finger Pulse & Doppler Test on myself, (& of course I had as I came up with the idea.) & Found a second fetal heartbeat?
Firstly, not being able to SEE anything on an abdominal scan means just that: they can't SEE anything.

What does this mean? Well, there are things that stop a clear image from being seen on an ultrasound scan because despite what you have been told ultrasounds are not perfect.

Gas in your belly, fat cells & scar tissue STOP the ultrasound waves from penetrating or seeing into your uterus properly. Funny that the doctors don't mention this to you because although google has had a lot of the truth scrubbed from it in recent years, it will tell you this.

I also have a tipped uterus & many women do. This is another reason a CP baby can't be seen on a scan because you often have to switch positions & the tech has to use different settings on the scan machine & even put a cushion under your bottom to be able to see deeply enough into the uterus to find the baby.

This will just not be done at all if your pregnancy tests are negative.

I personally had a lot of scar tissue during my CPs as I had a very bad c section with my first child that resulted in a huge amount of abdominal scaring, so it was even harder to visualise my CP baby during any scan but here's the thing; when your pregnancy tests are positive & you have a scan, the doctor or tech HAS to find a baby.

They do particular tests while looking in the uterus if your pregnancy tests are positive. For example, they measure the thickness of the uterus lining if your tests are positive & they are looking for a baby as they think this helps to date the pregnancy.

If you are CP, so have negative pregnancy tests & you have continued to have your monthly cycle, the scan might show a thin uterus lining. (You may also have a thin uterus lining if you have stopped having your cycle. See chapter three.)

If you have a thin uterus lining & negative pregnancy tests the doctor WILL NOT BE LOOKING FOR A BABY.

I repeat: IF YOUR PREGNANCY TESTS ARE NEGATIVE & YOUR UTERUS LINING IS THIN BECAUSE YOU ARE HAVING REGULAR CYCLES THE DOCTOR OR TECH PERFORMING YOUR SCAN IS NOT LOOKING FOR A BABY.
I can't stress this enough & yes; I have been there myself & spoken to many CP women all over the world during the last ten years who have had the same experience.

As I have said elsewhere, the medical cartel has instructed medical students very differently in the last twenty years or so to only trust medical tests & not to use common sense or logical deduction half as much as they used to.

It's quite tragic but understandable from a Gnostic point of view as the ontological or spiritual nature of over 70% of the population right now is that of false humans or demons & they are basically programmable robots or computers.

So even if they wanted to think correctly about a situation, they lack the ability to do so.

I understand that these Gnostic terms might be hard to accept, especially as many of us have been taught that medical schools only teach the brightest & the best, but this is just not the case anymore.

If it were the case, we wouldn't have such a huge CP problem worldwide, would we?

During a scan if your pregnancy tests are negative the doctor is looking for cysts, fibroids & tumours (more on this in chapter nine.) so when my abdominal scan at six months CP read that nothing could be seen I soon understood the reasons why after some research. If your scan report says that they can't find ether of your ovaries this is a HUGE indication that you are at least twenty weeks pregnant as ovaries cannot be seen on ultrasound IF the uterus is enlarged due to pregnancy. Obviously.

The tech will often tell you, as my scan tech told me, that you will need to be seen again because they couldn't see anything. What they don't tell you however is that they KNOW there is something there & they need to get to the bottom of it. If they, did you might think you were still pregnant despite negative pregnancy tests & they wouldn't want, you thinking that now would they?

Of course, as soon as your pregnancy tests are positive your baby is usually found on an abdominal scan because the medical professional will make you switch positions if your uterus is tilted & do everything they can do, to find that baby because the positive pregnancy test tells them that they have to.

This is not an extensive look at why a scan can be empty if you have one during a CP, but it gives you more than enough food for thought.

It's hard to believe you are pregnant after the great gods of science the medical professionals have declared you are not due to negative pregnancy tests & a so called empty ultrasound but you are actually SAFER believing you are pregnant during a CP despite all of this IF you have passed the Finger Pulse & Doppler Test by finding a fetal heartbeat of 120bpm or more on a doppler, whilst your own pulse is 60 to 90bpm taken at the same time.

As well as risking high blood pressure & preeclampsia ignoring a CP could make you believe that you are having reoccurring miscarriages when in fact nothing could be further from the truth.

Reoccurring miscarriage or CP?

One of the saddest things I've come across in over a decade whilst researching a cryptic pregnancy is women who think they are having reoccurring early miscarriages or chemical pregnancies when in fact they are having a CP.

Almost every month they are on the pregnancy & early miscarriage online groups in bits because they think they are having loss after loss after loss, & of course the medical cartel has no answers for them.

Let's break it down for a minute.

A chemical pregnancy is a very early miscarriage & happens around the time of your expected missed period. The woman begins to bleed & although the bleeding is often the same or LIGHTER than her normal cycle, she believes because her pregnancy tests have turned negative that she has lost the baby & of course this is the only explanation a doctor will give her.

Wait that sounds a bit like a cryptic pregnancy because CP women often continue a cycle but it's lighter. CP women also OFTEN have a few positive pregnancy tests one month then negative the next. This could be due to the high dose hook effect as we have said or the fact that as pregnancy progresses different forms of HCG are made. So, it follows that if most of the pregnancy tests on the market today just test for the early form of HCG, not every woman who is really pregnant is going to get a positive as their body will not be making the early form of HCG for very long.

Hello?

One thing that could rule out a chemical pregnancy is taking a pregnancy test once the bleeding has stopped. If it's positive she may be experiencing a CP & not any kind of miscarriage at all.

We have all heard of women who blithely tell anyone who will listen that they had a regular cycle throughout their pregnancy, but their doctor was never concerned because he said for them it was normal.

So, to rule out the fact that a woman who thinks she is having a chemical pregnancy is not:

  A. One of those pregnant women who continues a cycle each month during her pregnancy.

   Or B. having a cryptic pregnancy.

she must do a pregnancy test AFTER the bleeding has stopped.

  If it's positive, then she should go to the doctor for confirmation.

If the test is negative but she ether feels movement or just feels that something isn't right she should take the Finger Pulse & Doppler Test & if there is a second heartbeat of 120bpm or more whilst hers on the finger pulse is 60 to 90bpm, she is having a CP & she hasn't lost the baby at all.

Imagine the heartache she would avoid if she knew she hadn't had an early miscarriage & more importantly, wasn't having reoccurring early miscarriages each month. As let's face it, when you think about it, that's a bit of an impossibility right? How long does it take the average woman to conceive? At least a year now a days so how likely is it that a woman can get pregnant month after month after month & lose each foetus? I'm sure it does happen but it's not half as common as doctors would have us believe it is.

Very early reoccurring miscarriages & chemical pregnancies are a new thing & something I never ever heard about twenty years ago when I was pregnant with my first child.

So why is it seemingly everywhere now? I believe it is yet another thing the medical cartel have cooked up to try & hide the Truth about a CP. However, it's really easy to see through if you just use some basic common sense & skills of deduction.
So, understanding that reoccurring early miscarriages or chemicals could very well be a CP is a huge reason why ignoring a CP isn't wise as you could get stuck in the awful cycle of believing you are losing viable pregnancies when in fact nothing could be further from the truth.

A missed miscarriage or a CP?

I've known many women over the years who have gone through the devastation of a missed miscarriage. It is truly heart-breaking but supposing a missed miscarriage is not a miscarriage at all but a CP?

Surely everything should be ruled out by the medical cartel long BEFORE drugs are offered to make the woman miscarry, or a medical procedure is offered.

Let's examine the symptoms of a missed miscarriage or MM.

Bleeding, cramping & back pain are the only specific symptoms listed so it's extremely vague on purpose.

According to the NHS website the most common symptom is bleeding, but many CP women continue their cycle each month through their CP plus the NHS website states that:

Light bleeding is relatively common in the first trimester.

This is pure double speak & the medical cartel often do this. They contradict things to confuse & to try & hide the fact that they do not really have any proof you have had a MM unless they have actually SEEN a foetus that has definitely passed away on a scan.

Now IF you have been told you have had a MM because your baby looks small for dates, PLEASE have a long hard think about your next move & LISTEN TO YOUR GUT.

As discussed above, there are an awful lot of reasons why a baby can't be visualised properly on a scan so may look a lot smaller than it really is.

Sometimes it's just the way the baby is positioned. Let's not forget too that babies hate ultrasound so try to swim away from the probe. This of course makes the baby harder to see & measure correctly.

With my first child only twenty years ago you had a first scan at 14 weeks & very rarely before.

By week 14 babies can often be seen quite well but as with all babies, children & adults, a foetus in Utero will grow at its own rate so of course some may measure small for dates.
You need to ask yourself & the doctor, what is the standard measurement for a healthy foetus of the same gestation as yours & probably more importantly, HOW was that standard measurement arrived at because if you are a small slim woman, the measurements the doctors use for the average 14-week-old foetus might be from tall women who have a much larger build then you do.

If that's the case how any doctor with any real common sense can compare your 14-week baby's scan measurements with a foetus whose genetics will allow it to be much bigger than yours I just don't know.

So, if you have been told you have had a missed miscarriage because your baby looks small for dates and you are AT LEAST 14 weeks pregnant, WAIT & book a private scan in two or three week's & do NOT tell the tech that you have been told you are small for dates. Remember to tell them that you have irregular cycles so do NOT know the date of your last cycle. This way they might have the common sense to look for a baby larger than 14 weeks gestation, so have your scan & see what they tell you.

Remember patience is a virtue.

Why lie to the doctor or ultrasound tech you say?

Well let's face it, most doctors have been lying to CP women for years by telling them they are not PREGNANT because their pregnancy tests are negative BUT refusing to check for the baby's heartbeat, which is part of the actual diagnostic criteria for a false pregnancy.

To further illustrate this point, with one of my CP pregnancies (that tuned into a normal pregnancy quite quickly thankfully.) I went to my GP telling him I felt pregnant but had only had a faint positive. I was at least five months CP by then. I could tell the doctor wasn't stupid when he said, "If you really are past twenty weeks pregnant, we will find a fetal heartbeat." So, he got out his doppler & began to listen for a fetal heartbeat.

Sure, enough soon we could both hear the galloping of horses' sound of the baby's heartbeat, but we could ALSO hear & SEE the baby kicking & swiping at the doppler from outside of my belly!

As the doctor kept losing the heartbeat as my baby was moving so much, & I could of course feel this movement, he would quickly move the probe to try & find it again. The baby was too fast for him so finally he gave up & said I had to take the doctors pregnancy test.

I did & it was negative so of course the doctor said, "you are definitely not pregnant"

I laughed & replied, "But we both just heard the heartbeat & you were literally chasing the moving baby around my belly? What you blacked out & don't remember that doc?" He just said that the pregnancy test can't lie.

A sad situation as I actually thought he was one of the smart ones. I hadn't come up with the Finger Pulse & Doppler Test back then but if I had I would have insisted calmly that he did the test.

So as doctors have & do lie to CP women everyday what makes you think they can't lie to women & tell them they have had a MM & need surgery or drugs to start the miscarriage because the woman's body doesn't know she's had a miscarriage, so it needs help?

Of course, MM occur but if you have not seen a baby without a heartbeat on a scan then how can the doctor or anyone know for sure that the baby has passed? So always get a second & third & even fourth opinion or go for a private scan if you can afford it, after waiting it out a few weeks.

If you have been told you have had a MM long BEFORE you are 14 weeks pregnant always wait till 14 weeks, then demand another scan. The reason pregnant women were not offered a scan twenty years ago until they were at least 14 weeks was because the medical cartel was a little more honest back then so knew that a baby is rarely seen properly before week 14 specially if the woman has a tipped uterus & many women do.

As you can see, a CP can be mistaken for a chemical, reoccurring & a missed miscarriage, but knowledge is power. Always go with your intuition & never take the word of a doctor over your own gut just because they pretend to know more about your own body than you do.

9.
The fibroid dermoid cyst & Pregnancy of unknown location lies

In this chapter we will examine a brilliant old school medical textbook called The Mysteries of Human Reproduction: The Ovist Theory of Reproduction by Dr. Raymond W. Bernard published in 1959.

This book, along with many of the medical & Gnostic books I have used for my CP research over the years are almost impossible to get hold of now.

I wonder why?

Here is one of my favourite quotes from the book & if you are serious about CP research you might want to read the pdf online if you can't get hold of a hard copy, " it is now accepted by the medical profession that human ovum, under certain conditions, can parthenogenetically develop into a foetus within the body…while formally such foetuses (dermoid cysts,) were mistaken for tumours and considered pathological...If such parthenogenetic growths are not molested by surgery and if their development is not rendered abnormal by adverse parental emotional influences, they many develop into healthy living children."

In this chapter I will prove that because of negative pregnancy tests live healthy CP babies are often mistaken for fibroids & dermoid cysts & worse, once the surgeon or doctor realises this, the baby is almost never left alone to grow in the womb or given to its mother if it's full term, but ether stolen or killed.

I sadly know a woman personally who has been through this so let's first examine her harrowing story.

We met Alice in chapter six. She was the mother who had DNA tests done on her two very gifted children that proved she had self-conceived the children as they had no paternal DNA. Both children a girl & a boy, only had their mother's Maternal DNA.

In light of this fact & what we discovered in chapter four about a CP & divine birth, is it any wonder that CP mothers are often lied to & told their baby is just a fibroid for example?

It makes complete sense when you understand the greater Gnostic reality, that most of this world is run by humans with an evil demonic consciousness or fake humans whose nature it is to steal kill & destroy.

Sadly, the medical cartel is full of such beings these days so you must take off your rose-coloured glasses when dealing with most medical professionals as let's face it, if they really are so good & helpful you wouldn't be going through a CP you would have a confirmed pregnancy.

They would have used the Finger Pulse & Doppler Test to find your baby's heartbeat, or another medical test to find the fetal heartbeat as soon as you went to see them complaining of feeling pregnant yet having negative tests.

I first me Alice because I had seen her heart stopping YouTube video on one of the online CP groups & reached out to her.
She looked full term in the video & her big, obviously pregnant belly was rolling & MOVING the way a normal pregnant woman's belly rolls & moves once the baby is full term.

Having had normal pregnancies & CP pregnancies that turned normal, it was obvious to me that there was a baby in there. You really do not need a medical degree to recognise a full-term baby moving & rolling in a pregnant woman's belly & no, gas cannot POSSIBLY MOVE & KICK in that way. Plain old common sense should tell you that.

Sadly, her doctor had told her because her pregnancy tests were negative, she couldn't be pregnant & no other tests were offered to rule out pregnancy.
She had instead been told that she had a fibroid that often rolled & moved in her belly & usually to music.

By the time I spoke to Alice she had been CP for over two years & wanted out. Her belly was very big & she just couldn't take it anymore so when her doctor offered to operate & remove the fibroid, she had no real choice so agreed.

This is why there is a lot of information in chapter five of this book about how not to allow yourself to put on enough weight to look pregnant UNTIL your pregnancy tests turn positive & you are confirmed by the medical cartel during a CP.
I was still going clubbing throughout my last CP. I made sure not to look pregnant (although I definitely weighed more.) and nobody would have guessed that I was.

If you do allow yourself to grow a pregnant belly, like Alice, you might feel you have no choice due to the emotional & physical stress of your size, but to go along with a doctor's wrong diagnosis of your CP baby & agree to the same kind of operation.

Alice will probably spend the rest of her life regretting agreeing to having her fibroid removed.

On the day before her operation, she made the doctor promise that if he saw a baby, he would stop the operation & if it were full term, as she was way past nine months CP, he would deliver it.

The doctor simply replied, "of course Alice but as you are having a delusional pregnancy, we won't see a baby so please don't worry about that."

She was put to sleep for the removal of her fibroid but when she woke up, she was on the maternity ward with mothers who had just given birth. She frantically asked the midwife who came to do her stats what had happened. Had she had a baby? where was the baby?!

The nurse seemed frightened & finally told her it was more than her jobs worth to tell Alice what she knew but that she would ask her doctor to come & speak to her.

Alice had had two normal births before & not only did she feel like she had just given birth she was also bleeding in the same way a woman would after giving birth.

She also noticed a painful vaginal laceration the same kind she had when she gave birth to her first child when the doctor had used forceps to get the baby out.

She begged & pleaded to see her doctor, but he couldn't be contacted.

The very next day that doctor resigned.

She told me, "I had definitely given birth, there were no incisions in my abdomen as they said there would have been to take the so-called fibroid out & I know what it feels like after giving birth. They stole my baby! I said it again & again until one of the nurses came to calm me down. I think they gave me something to make me sleep, but I knew they'd taken my child & lied to cover it up. Before I was discharged one of the midwives on the maternity ward, I'd been put on came to tell me that medical negligence had taken place & yes as far as she knew I had given birth to a live baby, but the doctor had taken it. I got a hold of my medical notes & it said nothing about a baby just that a large fibroid had been removed from my uterus. If it weren't for that I would have called the police & reported my doctor for kidnapping the baby, but I had no PROOF I'd even been pregnant let alone given birth!"

The last time I spoke to Alice, she told me the original midwife was willing to testify in court that she knew Alice had given birth & not had a fibroid removed at all but of course, it was going to be their word against the doctors.

If you were a judge, who would you believe? An upstanding medical doctor or a poor single mother?
Sadly, it's a no brainer as so often in this world, money & prestige always win & there is rarely justice for the good or the hurting.

In chapter five of The Mysteries of Human Reproduction Dr Raymond W. Bernard reveals these astounding facts about parthenogenesis & dermoid cysts, "It is not generally known by the laity that medical literature contains abundant records of cases in which there have been removed from virgins, underdeveloped embryos, and foetuses in various stages of growth. There is no explanation to account for this curious phenomenon except that, through the operation of unknown forces, a human egg has been caused to parthenogenetically develop into an embryo in the body of a virgin. The most significant aspect of such cases is that they constitute an indisputable part of medical practice and hence cannot be denied even if their significance is not generally discussed or admitted by the medical profession."

Yet there you were thinking your doctor always tells the truth.

We know from my findings in chapter four that CP women have often conceived by parthenogenesis & it is my belief that the spiritual ontology of a woman is the reason for this. True Beings have more of a chance to conceive in this way because their Spirit was created by the Absolute, so they have the divine Energy to do so. As we are in the very last days there are very few True Beings left on the planet so obviously, parthenogenesis is quite rare.

As Dr Bernard points out, live healthy foetuses are often mistaken for dermoid cysts & fibroids because Alice is not the first CP woman I have spoken too, who has sadly lost their CP baby in this horrifying way.

But are these honest mistakes? Can doctors really be that THICK? Or is there something more nefarious going on?

He goes on to say, "should a dermoid cyst (or fibroid.) reach full development, we would have a virgin (& a CP.) produced child. It is probable then that many so called dermoid cysts might do so if not operatively interfered with, under the erroneous belief that human parthenogenesis is not possible. In fact, there is no evidence that all dermoid cysts (or so-called fibroids.) are pathological. Some may be perfectly normal parthenogenetic embryos who were needlessly removed by operation, under the belief that they would never develop into living children. (Because the mother had negative pregnancy tests?) However, the virgin mothers of England." A reference to Emmimarie Jones whose daughter Monica was found to have been conceived by parthenogenesis by British doctors in the 1950's, see chapter four. "Who developed such embryos to full term as normal children proved that this is possible." words in brackets mine.

So, if dermoid cysts & fibroids are not pathological are you beginning to join the dots with CP babies? Now do you understand why these so-called fibroids are often removed? The Truth can be stranger than fiction.

If you, a CP woman have been told by your doctor that you need a fibroid, dermoid cyst or noncancerous tumour removed from your uterus it may well be a live healthy CP baby so be very careful that Alice's story does not become your own.

If you have had a scan during your CP or ever read in your medical notes the word teratoma in reference to something that is in your uterus, please understand that this is another medical word for dermoid cyst. In Chambers Dictionary the word literally means, foetus or embryonic growth.

Now we don't know that in every case a fibroid or a dermoid cyst is actually a live, healthy CP baby but we DO KNOW that doctors have been known to lie & cover up a lot about cryptic pregnancies.

Not only are they covering up the fact that most CP women ARE really pregnant by refusing to honesty listen for a fetal heartbeat, they are also lying & covering up CP babies being seen on scans. I know as this has happened to me.

So, when they tell you that you are not pregnant, but you have a large cyst, or fibroid or a noncancerous tumour in your uterus or on your fallopian tube (how could anything actually grow ON a fallopian tube? Where would the blood supply come from? Wouldn't the tube burst?!) are they REALLY telling you the truth or are they lying to your face?

Only you can be the judge of that. Just go with your intuition & don't end up in a sea of regret like Alice & many CP women like her. Nothing can bring your CP baby back once the medical cartel has taken it saying it was a fibroid, cyst, or noncancerous tumour as you have NO proof you were even pregnant in the first place if your pregnancy tests were negative. It's your word against the medical cartel.

I am not the first person in history to point this out as Dr Bernard also said regarding dermoid cysts, "Some maybe perfectly normal parthenogenetic embryos who were NEEDLESSLY removed by operation." Do not let this be your CP baby.

The term pregnancy of unknown location is often casually & erroneously used by the medical cartel to describe what happens when your pregnancy tests finally turn positive & your cycle stops during a CP, but your baby cannot be found on ultrasound. This situation is so common, even with normal non-CP pregnancies that it almost always results in one in four MEDICAL miscarriages according to statistics.

Why?

Because the medical cartel, using the blind & foolish trust most people put in them, often convince women to KILL a healthy unborn baby because they insist it can't be seen on ultrasound when in fact a clear ultrasound view of the whole uterus is extremely limited for many women.

As a result, unborn babies, wanted babies are being murdered needlessly & somebody needs to speak up.

Well, here I am.

This is a frighting situation & something I have been through personally so let me take you there.

I had been single for a long time, around three years just happily living my life & doing my thing when I met this guy who seemed to make time stop.

Lightning bolts, heart beating out of your chest, serious can't eat can't sleep stuff. It was the real Robert palmer deal. (Lit 80s song called Addicted to Love performed by British Artist Robert palmer.) & It was mutual.

After about a year of the kind of romance you think only ever happens on Netflix until it happens to you, my cycle stopped, but as I had been following my own advice in chapter three, I honestly didn't think much of it until one day three months later I took a pregnancy test because I was feeling really sick in the mornings & then three more. They were all positive. This wasn't a CP pregnancy & I knew the date of conception as my lover owned an international company so had been in & out of the county for over three months & we hadn't been able to get together.

I waited for at least a month to make sure I had no bleeding & took a test each day to make sure it stayed positive & then went to the doctor for confirmation. They sent me to the midwife & strangely she didn't ask me to do a pregnancy test. I had brought along four of my different brands positive tests & she seemed cool with that.

They booked me in for a scan the very next day as according to my cycle I was almost twenty weeks. I actually didn't look it because CP or not, I made an effort to stay slim like Patrica Carter in chapter five because my body my choice shouldn't only be applied to women who want abortions. If I want to stay as slim as I can during pregnancy I can & so, can you. It's your body plus it's a million times healthier than putting on too much weight.

I knew it was too good to be true when the scan technician put the probe on my belly & after a few seconds said simply, "I can't see a pregnancy." she then tried the internal, still nothing.

This is when I began to realise how deep this rabbit hole really goes.

She was saying that the lining of my uterus was thin so I couldn't be pregnant. Eye roll times a hundred as we know from chapter three that historically, many women have had healthy pregnancies & babies, yet they have never had a cycle. Having a monthly cycle & therefore a thick uterus lining has little to do with healthy ovulation & pregnancy, it is just one of the medical cartel's fairy tales, please see chapter three. My lover's ontology was obviously NOT that of a fake human or a demon so the fact that the lining was less than 3mm thick only further proved to me my own theory on menstruation in chapter three.

I knew I was pregnant as although just under twenty weeks I had tried my own Finger Pulse & Doppler Test & had found a second heartbeat of 165 on the doppler whilst mine on a finger pulse was 71bpm.

Plus, I had positive tests plus no cycle & definitely no pain, bleeding, or spotting.
I had also been feeling movement.

 The tech then asked for a urine sample because she wanted me to run a pregnancy test, but as she had made me empty my bladder for the internal ultrasound only ten minutes before I couldn't pee.
I wasn't going to drink loads of water & try to pee, although she had asked me to do this, in case my urine would be too dilute to get a positive test.

I wasn't falling for that old chestnut.

So, she printed out her scan report & sent me to get bloods taken to see what my blood HCG numbers were. Kill me now I thought.

 Below on page sixty-four is my actual scan report & surprise, as I have said before if a doctor or scan tech says they can't SEE anything on your scan it literally means that they can't SEE anything because SOMETHING is blocking the view!

The important part circled in green & marked part A says: ultrasound view RESTRICTED by overlaying bowel gas & previous surgery. (I have had more than one c section plus a tummy tuck.)

& Part B circled in red says: pregnancy site uncertain & worse, as you can see just below part B, the so-called diagnosis was the dreaded PUL or pregnancy of unknown location.

But wait a minute doc, HOLD ON, HOLD ON, HOLD ON! didn't you just say on the report that the view of the uterus was RESTRICTED?

Yes, you did. It's right there in black & white.

So, what does the world restricted mean? Simply put the word means unable to see clearly. So, they ADMIT that they couldn't SEE my uterus clearly so LOGICALLY, they should do everything to SEE the uterus clearly BEFORE labelling me with a PUL.

Come on now.

But of course, the medical cartel do not operate with good old fashioned common sense these days oh no. They would rather assume it's ectopic (another false diagnosis often given to CP women once their pregnancy has turned normal sadly.) Or tell me I have had their old favourite, a missed miscarriage.

Again, a missed miscarriage is where your body doesn't know the baby has died so the medical cartel has to gallop in on its twisted white horse & give you drugs or worse, an evacuation to KILL YOUR OFTEN HEALTHY UNBORN BABY.

You couldn't make it up.

They took my bloods & of course the doctor later called me sounding very excited, (yes most of them are that sick.) to say I'd definitely had a miscarriage from the blood results.
I knew they were wrong because I had taken another pregnancy test when I got home, and it was a clear big fat positive again. So, I said, "ok doc, what now because I'm not bleeding & I have no pain so where the miscarriage is?"

He said I would probably bleed at some point & if not the baby would be REABSORBED.

Yet I KNEW & the midwife had confirmed to me only the day before that I was TWENTY WEEKS!

So how can a twenty-week foetus be reabsorbed?!

I swear some of these so-called medical professionals must think that most pregnant women came down in the last snowstorm.

To his credit, my new GP was very understanding, (he was old school.) specially as after a week I'd had no bleeding or pain & had taken more pregnancy tests all of which were of course positive. He kept trying to call the hospital to arrange a follow up because he actually seemed to think, as anyone with half a brain cell would, that their diagnosis was completely mad.

So, I did what anyone with an ounce of common sense would do & waited until I was 24 weeks & then paid for a private 4D scan. Of course, the baby was found high up in my uterus safe & healthy measuring right along with being around 25 weeks gestation. I had known all along the baby was in my uterus but HIGH UP & BEHIND MY INTESTINES as they were stuck to my uterus due to my previous c sections & tummy tuck. I had obviously told the midwife & the original scan tech all of this but bless them, neither of these women were the brightest tools in the box.

I am now suing the NHS for damages & the litigation is ongoing.

So PUL, pregnancy of unknown location in simple logical terms means: A PREGNANCY THAT CAN NOT BE SEEN ON A
SCAN, NOT BECAUSE IT IS NOT THERE BUT BECAUSE MOST OF THE MEDICAL CARTEL ARE BLIND UNCOMPREHENDING ROBOTS WHO WILL NOT ADMIT THAT SCANS HAVE MANY LIMITATIONS WHEN VISUALISING

THE UTERUS. This will be discussed in greater detail in The Cryptic Pregnancy Files volume two.

To illustrate supposing we are standing at the train station waiting for my brother to meet us but it's dark & raining hard. My brother texts to say he is five minutes away. And so, I tell you,

"Chill, he's like five minutes away so you'll see him in a minute." You don't buy it so four minutes later you say,

"I'm looking Neo, but I can't see him, and I've been looking for ages! Let's go to the beach. He is obviously at the beach because I can't see him."

So, I'm like, "what? Wait, how is the BEACH the same as the station? Are you SERIOUSLY telling me because you can't see him through all of this rain & darkness, he is NOT THERE at all?"

Suddenly my brother Joe taps me on the shoulder laughing, "couldn't you guys see me! I was waving at you as I was walking up. I could see you guys, but you couldn't see me. I guess you couldn't VISUALISE ME CLEARLY through the dark & all this crazy weather. My bad. Let's go!"
So, was Joe at the beach? Nope. He was close to the station the whole time we just couldn't see him through the rain & the darkness.

TO SAY THAT BECAUSE THE DARK & BAD WEATHER OBSCURED HIM FROM VIEW, HE WAS SOMEWHERE ELSE COMPLETELY WOULD MAKE YOU VERY STUPID INDEED SADLY.

This is the exact kind of illogical madness the medical cartel try & feed you when they say they can't see your unborn baby on a scan yet many things like bowel gases or a tipped uterus are making a clear view IMPOSSIBLE.

You do not HAVE to do everything the doctors tell you know? This is not Simon says. Stay away from them, don't do their silly blood tests & if you have no pain, do not start bleeding & your tests are STILL positive pay for a private scan in two or three weeks.
Most women do not have the kind of abdominal adhesions I have so their babies can be found on an ordinary abdominal scan if they would just have some good old-fashioned PATIENCE.

As this is a huge problem that effects not only CP women after the CP turns normal, but many women with normal pregnancies too, somebody needs to throw a light on these disgusting medical murders & the cover up so it might as well be me.

In the next chapter, we will examine how to deal with doctors during a CP & once your CP turns normal so you can always have the upper hand when dealing with the medical cartel.

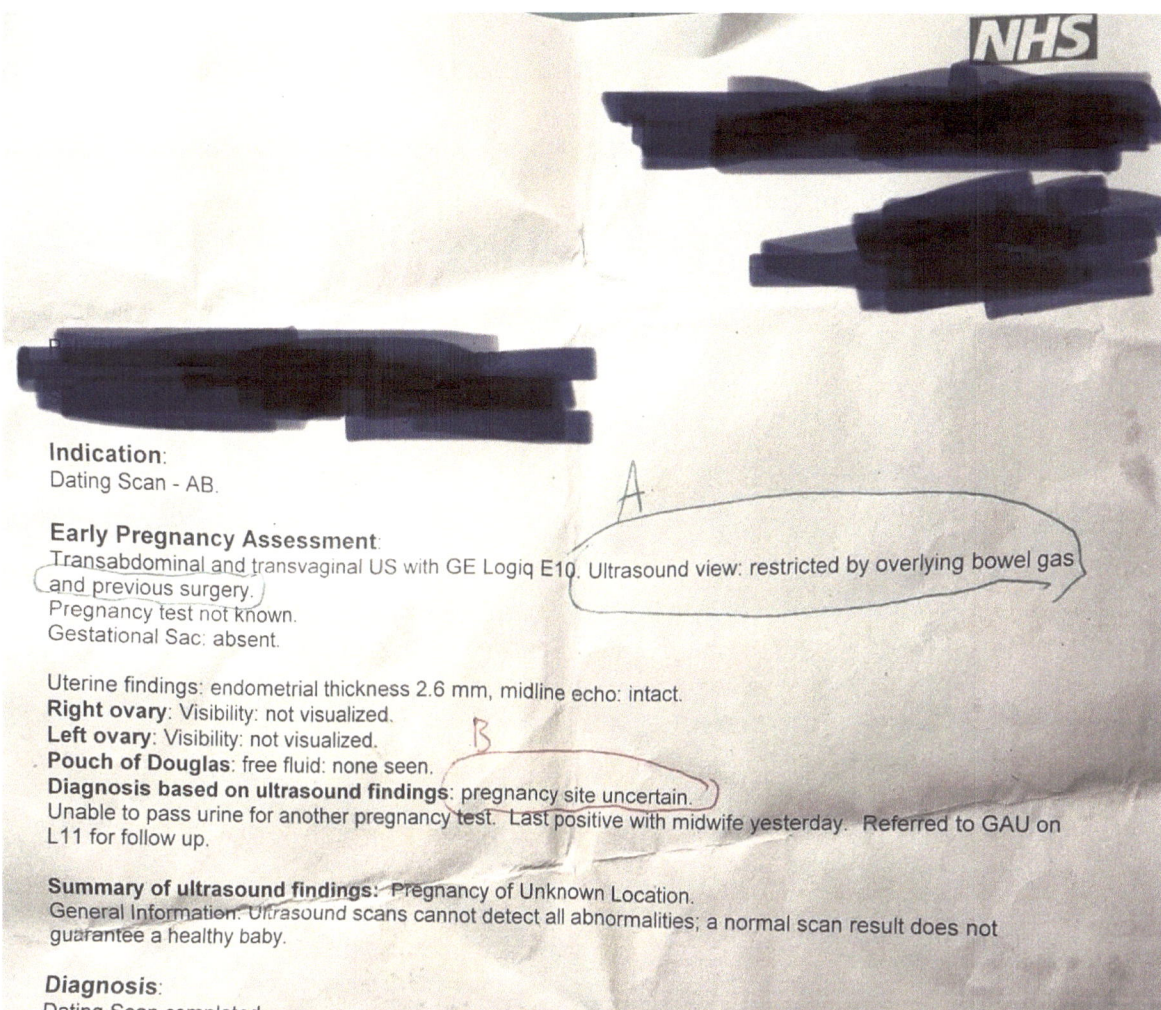

Indication:
Dating Scan - AB.

Early Pregnancy Assessment:
Transabdominal and transvaginal US with GE Logiq E10. Ultrasound view: restricted by overlying bowel gas and previous surgery.
Pregnancy test not known.
Gestational Sac: absent.

Uterine findings: endometrial thickness 2.6 mm, midline echo: intact.
Right ovary: Visibility: not visualized.
Left ovary: Visibility: not visualized.
Pouch of Douglas: free fluid: none seen.
Diagnosis based on ultrasound findings: pregnancy site uncertain.
Unable to pass urine for another pregnancy test. Last positive with midwife yesterday. Referred to GAU on L11 for follow up.

Summary of ultrasound findings: Pregnancy of Unknown Location.
General Information: Ultrasound scans cannot detect all abnormalities; a normal scan result does not guarantee a healthy baby.

Diagnosis:
Dating Scan completed.

10. How to deal with medical professionals during a CP

Let's be honest now, the medical profession has always had a twisted view of its own self-importance but today it's worse than ever as science it seems, is the new world religion. Just read Rupert Sheldrakes eye opening book on the subject The Science Delusion.

Nobody wants to be seen to consider anything outside of the scientific box but what people fail to realise is that most of so-called science is just a theory or an unproven idea.

Just like epigenesis is JUST a theory & Professor Jacques Loeb's Ovist theory that states a human female ovum can generate into a foetus without a male sperm present is another theory of conception, but it suited the powers that be to only promote epigenesis.

Many medical theories are promoted that are almost certainly questionable at best. The idea that pregnancy tests can't produce false negatives is quite obviously wrong as the high dose hook effect proves this, but you won't hear any medical professionals admit this to you any time soon.

When examining a cryptic pregnancy, the suffering, pain, humiliation & frustration a CP woman feels almost every second of every day is purely & only BECAUSE OF THE MEDICAL DOCTORS lack of integrity, honestly & quite frankly, intellect.

Please let that sink in for a moment.

If the medical world actually did what their own medical literature states they should do if they think a woman is having a false pregnancy, they will listen honestly for a fetal heartbeat because a false or delusional pregnancy can only be confirmed with A. a negative pregnancy test & B. the complete absence of a fetal heartbeat.

You can't have one without the other I'm afraid but just because it suits them over 99.9% of doctors WRONGLY believe, for whatever reason, that if a woman's pregnancy tests are negative & she STILL feels pregnant, she is having a false pregnancy.

Yet there are many peers reviewed medical articles about the high dose hook effect online & doctors must know this.

So, if they know that a woman can be pregnant with negative tests due to the high dose hook effect for example, why don't they do the common sense & logical next step & rule out a fetal heartbeat?

Your guess is as good as mine to be honest, but I have spoken to a few doctors over the years about this in a very calm respectful manner of course, & they all seem to get very nervous, stumble over their words & change the subject for some reason.

It is beyond bizarre.

Please look up a false pregnancy in any medical literature, textbook, google or on WEBMD & you will find that the doctor absolutely needs to make sure there is NO FETAL HEARTBEAT if a woman is having a false pregnancy.

So how do you deal with doctors when going through a CP?

You must be as wise as serpents & as gentle as doves & outsmart your doctors as much, if not more so then he has you because he is making your life a misery purely because he won't do one simple Finger Pulse & Doppler Test. So, use his tools of denial to your advantage.
How?

Let's start by examining the case study of a CP woman I know well who went to see her doctor around three months CP.
Kathrine was thirty-two, from London & already a mother to a happy healthy six-year-old daughter.
She wasn't exactly over the moon with the prospect of another child so soon as she was studying for a law degree part time so was considering an abortion. So, when she missed her cycle & her pregnancy test was negative, she didn't worry too much. She took another test when she would have been eight weeks pregnant & it was positive. Wanting to explore her options she went straight to her local sexual health walk in clinic hoping to be given information about an early abortion but when the obviously disengaged nurse asked her to take a pregnancy test it came back negative. Kathrine was relived but confused. The nurse said she had probably just had an early miscarriage & to go see her GP in a few weeks if her cycle hadn't arrived & ask for pills to start it.

Kathrine left knowing that she wouldn't do that. She wasn't trying for a baby as she was on off with her music industry suit lover & knew he wouldn't want to settle down & have a baby with her although she was falling for him.

She felt she had dodged a bullet & was fully expecting her cycle to begin any day as her belly felt heavy & strange.

By twelve weeks she couldn't take it anymore. Her belly was swelling, she was hungrier, she felt sick first thing in the morning & had all the pregnancy symptoms she had with her daughter except that her pregnancy tests where completely negative!

She was so angry with herself as she had spent a small fortune on different pregnancy tests by then.

However, Kathrine believed the negative pregnancy tests, took appetite suppressants to help curb her hunger & tried to forget about it.

When Kathrine would have been fifteen weeks pregnant, she felt baby flutters.

She had been washing up after dinner & almost dropped a plate when she felt it.
It was an unmistakable tickling in her belly, just the same as it had been with her daughter.

At that moment she knew two things: She was REALLY pregnant despite her negative pregnancy tests & she would keep the baby & her music industry lover would have to like it or lump it, but she figured he'd come round eventually as they had talked about kids.

She went to see her GP first thing in the morning & after explaining that she was really pregnant because she was feeling movement despite her negative tests, she was a bit annoyed when he seemed not to hear her but just asked her to provide a urine sample.

As the doctor dipped the pregnancy test strip in her cup, she held her breath but of course it was negative again.

"You are not Pregnant Kathrine. You may have a cyst. Let me give you some meds to start your cycle &."

"Thanks, but no thanks doctor, I am feeling regular FETAL MOVEMENT Just like I did with my daughter & I obviously know what it feels like. Can't you do a scan or listen for a heartbeat on a doppler like the midwives do or even just feel my belly! It's very hard & look…."

"No Kathrine that won't be necessary." The doctor cut her off. He wasn't even looking at her but typing fast with his hard blue eyes fixed on his computer screen. "Now if you keep insisting you are pregnant when your pregnancy tests are negative, I may have to call the mental health team & child social services."

"What! You are joking right?! I've never had any mental health issues & my daughter is fine, what has this even got to do with my child? Plus, I am NOT delusional! God, I'm studying for a law degree
so, I'm far too busy to be making things up!" By now she was quite upset but thankfully Kathrine was in my CP Facebook group & at that moment remembered me saying in one of my articles that you must remain very calm when dealing with doctors during a CP & you must learn to outsmart them.

So, Kathrine took a deep breath & taking hold of her rising emotion simply said, "ok, ok. You might be right. I can't be pregnant if the test is negative." (She wanted to roll her eyes but held back. She knew about the high dose hook effect. Obviously, her doctor didn't.) I'm sure my cycle will start soon. Thanks!" & She was wise enough to leave the doctor's office asap.

I spoke to Kathrine a lot over the next few weeks. She was lucky as being only fifteen weeks CP she had only put on a few pounds & knew instinctively that she definitely didn't want to look pregnant without a doctor's confirmation so as hard as it was, she continued to watch what she ate but made sure to eat a lot of protein to avoid high blood pressure & PE.

Things were going well in her relationship & she was smart enough to keep her CP/ pregnancy from her lover. Summer holiday were coming up & her daughter was due to go & stay with her grandmother for a few weeks, so I told Kathrine to take some time & maybe go away with her lover & try to forget about her CP.

I knew that the positive Energy & Life force that comes from being with a guy you're really in love with, as long as you are both of the same consciousness, could work wonders for her CP & even turn her pregnancy tests positive. Remember everything is about Energy.
She took my advice & continued to take a pregnancy test every week despite the negatives. She was halfway there as thankfully; her cycle hadn't started again.

Just after Kathrine was eighteen weeks CP & obviously feeling regular movement, she had a clearly positive pregnancy test. She went out & brought five other name brands just to be sure & they were all clear positives just like that!

Now she had to deal with her doctor but understandably, after how awful he had been to her at the last appointment she really didn't want to see him, yet she didn't want to wait to change doctors as it would take ages to get an appointment with a new doctor.

As her pregnancy tests where so positive & because she was under thirty-five told her to go to the hospital, complaining of pain in her belly & to see what they would come up with.

She laughed when I told her & simply said, "ok Neo. Let's play the doctors at their own game this time!"

I'll never forget the triumphant email I received from her a few days later. It read, "hi Neo, well I did what you said & it worked out better than I expected! So amazing how differently doctors treat you when you have that all important second line in seconds on a pregnancy test performed in front of them!

"So anyway, like we said, I went to the hospital complaining of pain in my belly & told them no I had not had a proper cycle for at least four months & no I had not thought to take a pregnancy test.
Yes, I obviously seemed a bit thick to them as I could tell they were already thinking I was a silly woman who was pregnant but hadn't bothered to test, but as you said it was important that the medical professionals thought they had figured out what was happening with me before they
 thought I had & it made sense. If I had gone in saying, I've been feeling pregnant for months! I feel the baby move all the time, but my tests have been negative until now! They probably would have thought I was crazy like my GP did & called the mental health team. Why are doctors so brain washed that they really think anyone who doesn't agree with them has to have serious mental health issues?

"Anyway, they asked me for my urine sample, dipped the pregnancy test & bang there it was a big fat positive! So, they said really gently as if it wasn't news I was wanting or expecting, you are pregnant Kathrine so let's do a scan to make sure everything's ok.

"My head was spinning. All those weeks of knowing I was pregnant but afraid to go back to the doctor for help because he tried to imply, I was crazy for asking him to listen for a second heartbeat after my negative test & here the doctor was telling me I was definitely pregnant!

"I hoped & prayed they would realise by the scan that I was eighteen weeks along, but I said nothing & let them do their thing.

Well, they dated the baby as being fifteen weeks & told me I'm having a boy!

Needless to say, I'm changing my GP for my antenatal care."

And who can blame her?

The other side to this is what if you don't want to continue your CP pregnancy? How can you get an abortion if your pregnancy tests are negative & a doctor won't believe you? I had been thinking this over quite a bit when a woman emailed me from California as she wanted to share her CP story with me.
Frankie worked in TV & really didn't want a baby let alone a long stressful CP. She had missed three cycles so although her tests were negative, at around twelve weeks CP she went to the abortion clinic & lied by saying she had had a positive pregnancy test & thought she was around three months pregnant.
What I didn't know until she told me was that you do NOT have to take a pregnancy test at an abortion clinic, they just take your word that you have had a positive test. They also scan you before your procedure to check how far along you are. When Frankie saw her baby for the first time on the ultrasound, she cried saying she would definitely not be having the abortion.
She wanted her baby & knew she would somehow work her career around it.

So, this got me thinking: what if you are at least twelve weeks CP & you can't take it anymore but WANT your baby? Where is the one place you can go where they won't perform a pregnancy test on you but WILL give you an honest abdominal ultrasound for free to make sure of your dates?

An abortion clinic.

Now this isn't for the faint hearted as if you really want to be a mother you might not want to go to a place like that but if you can just pretend you want an abortion until they give you a scan & you see your baby, you can suddenly change your mind & ask the doctor for a copy of your scan report & a letter for your doctor explaining how far along you are & that you wish to continue with the pregnancy. Yes, it may be a controversial way to get your pregnancy confirmed without a positive test but it's definitely an option.
Once you have that scan report you honestly won't have to fiddle about doing a pregnancy test with your doctor or midwife when you go & book in for your antenatal care.

What if you're CP & you're over thirty-five?

As a CP can last for years you could be well over thirty-five when your pregnancy turns normal.

This is a very difficult situation as because it's so hard to get pregnant these days most of the medical cartel stick to their erroneous religious belief that only women under thirty-five can possibly get pregnant. Remember many women self-conceive their CP baby so what is impossible with man is possible with God.

Of course, you can't tell the medical cartel any of this so stay away from doctors if you are in this age group as much as possible as even if you go in when your cycle stops & tests turn positive, they may tell you that you are in menopause so that explains your cycle stopping & worse, that pregnancy test are often positive during menopause, yet women are not really pregnant at all.

You couldn't make up the lies & half-truths the medical cartel come up with to try & hide the Truth about a CP, especially with older women but it's true. Just look this up.

If they won't believe you are pregnant when your test is positive with the doctor's pregnancy test & your cycle has stopped pay for a private abdominal scan. If you are at least nine months CP, tell them you have very irregular cycles, so you are not sure when you last had a cycle, but it was at LEAST five   months ago.

Tell the scan tech you didn't think to test for pregnancy as you feel fine & haven't put on much weight (hopefully this is true if you are past nine months CP for your own sake.) but you have taken some pregnancy tests & they are ALL positive. Be sure to bring the tests with you to show the tech or doctor & be willing to take a new pregnancy test there & then if they insist you must as yes, they can be that dim if they want to be I'm afraid. (Twenty years ago, when I had my first pregnancy confirmed I just took in my ONE positive pregnancy test, the only test I had taken, showed it to my GP & said, doctor I think I'm pregnant. The doctor took one look at my positive pregnancy test & said, congratulations! Let me book you in for your fourteen-week scan. And that was that! You really had to be there back in the day to believe it because things have changed so much.)

So, when you have your scan, they will know you have positive tests, & your cycle hasn't been around for months. (Make sure to drink plenty of water before an abdominal scan because this makes the baby easier to see as pushes your uterus up & avoid fizzy drinks, as they create bowel gas.) This helps them to look for a BIGGER baby than they would of you admitted your cycle had recently stopped. As you have to do the thinking FOR the medical cartel even when your CP turns normal because we are in a FIGHT for our lives & a fight for our CP child's life make no mistake.

Now the most important thing you must tell your scan tech when you pay for a private scan if you are over thirty-five & your CP has turned normal is that you are ten years younger than you really are.

So, if you are say, forty-four, tell them you are thirty-four & take ten years off of your birthday if they ask for the date. Why? Because the medical cartel can & do tell CP women over a particular age, even after their pregnancy tests are positive, that they have a FIBROID or noncancerous TUMOUR instead of a baby inside their belly on a scan & you know that this is often pure BS from the textbook medical evidence we have just examined in chapter nine.

Now because when you pay for a scan the tech doesn't have or need your medical records you will be fine taking ten years off of your age so they can find your baby.

A dear friend of mine Agnes who lives in Jamaican was forty-six when her six-year CP finally turned normal.

She went to her GP with her positive pregnancy test & he laughed at her saying she was just in menopause & women in menopause often get positive pregnancy tests! So, this can happen sadly.
Once your baby has been found on the scan & they have written your scan report & a letter for your doctor innocently look at your scan information & say, "hey doc it seems you have my age wrong. My birthday is ..." & give them your

real birthday & watch their face drop! It really will be a picture specially if you are say, forty-six like Agnes & told them you were thirty-six!

However, mistakes in patient names & birthdates often happen so you must make sure that they think they just misheard your age & your birthday was simply written down wrong.

The best thing? They can't change your scan report once it's done & your baby is found. They will just have to change your age on the scan report & then you can go to your own doctor as a winner because not only did you outsmart the medical cartel, you will soon be holding your CP baby as your pregnancy would have been confirmed not only with your positive pregnancy tests but your private scan report too.

I have a CP TikTok account called @neobrownoffical & some people have found it quite helpful as I post shorts on basic CP topics. A few of the videos have gone viral so they attract a lot of comments. One woman told me recently that she thought she had a cryptic pregnancy as she had felt pregnant on & off for months BUT hadn't taken a test as her cycle continued as normal, so she didn't think she needed to take a pregnancy test. She went for a scan for something else completely & the scan tech told her she was not only pregnant but full term & in labour! She said she had no pain at all & was completely amazed to say the least.

However, this was twenty-five years ago. So, as I have shown, the medical cartel are not half as logical & honest as they used to be, so I wasn't surprised her baby was found back then.

There must be some exceptions to the rule today so if you are at least five months CP & really can't take it anymore & your CP hasn't turned normal, you could try booking an abdominal scan & just say you've been having abdominal pain & irregular cycles. The baby is sadly unlikely to be found because everything is about the positive pregnancy test with the medical cartel these days but it's definitely worth a try. As long as you don't mention you've been feeling pregnant, they might be honest and find it.

No matter what age you are when your pregnancy tests turn positive & how long you have been CP do try to avoid pregnancy blood tests. These are often used in early pregnancy to try & convince the

mother because her HCG might not be in the normal range (yet all humans are different so what might be a normal HCG range for you might be very low or very high for another woman.) she must have her bloods drawn every few days & if the HCG isn't rising fast enough, she should agree to abort the baby asap. I've noticed this seems to happen often in America for some reason.

This is an evil & disgusting abuse of power by the medical cartel as most women trust their doctor & are brainwashed into being doubtful about the health of their tiny foetus just because its HCG numbers are not impressive enough for the doctor. Are some of these doctors Satanists because it seems many will say anything to convince a healthy woman into aborting her much wanted baby.

It does make you wonder.

Bottom line: don't fall for such a cheap trick. Respectfully decline pregnancy blood HCG testing specially if you have had a CP that's turned normal.
I knew one CP woman from one of the online groups who had been CP for at least six months & she actually looked six months pregnant. A few weeks later her cycle stopped & her tests where positive but because her doctor did her HCG blood test, they said she was actually SIX WEEKS PREGNANT.

Well, we all knew she was at least six months & so did she but what could she do but go along with what the doctor said? At least he wasn't asking her to abort the baby because her HCG was only showing six weeks gestation.

CP babies often produce HCG at much lower & slower levels so it's really not worth risking the HCG blood test. This relatively new idea of testing blood HCG in pregnancy every five minutes I believe should be banned unless there is an EXTREMELY good reason for it.

What if you have been to your doctor for help so many times during a CP that when your tests turn positive you fear they won't confirm you?

Sadly, this is a very valid fear for women who have been CP for a year or more yet have been bold enough to demand abdominal scans & even X-rays from their doctor to find out what exactly is going on inside their body, because when you push your doctor during a CP he will rarely crack & listen for a fetal heartbeat or perform the Finger Pulse & Doppler Test.

Oh no. He is likely to get angry & send you for mental health treatment as of course if you dare to disagree more than once with the great high priest of the medical cartel the GP doctor, much like in the Salem witch trials you are labelled crazy & delusional when back then you would have been labelled a crazy witch.

An X-ray, CT or MRI scan can indeed find a CP baby but AGAIN unless your radiologist has been told to look for a pregnancy because your pregnancy tests are positive & they can't visualise the baby correctly on a scan for example, they will more often than not conveniently MISS the baby EVEN IF THEY SEE ONE.

Such is the medical cartels blatant deceit towards women going through a cryptic pregnancy.

To illustrate my friend Gemma was forty-two & being way past nine months CP paid for an expensive 4D baby scan telling them she had a round mass in her stomach, but her doctor said it wasn't urgent as she wasn't in much pain. So, the clinic agreed to do the 4D scan. During the scan, the tech didn't say a word. They just gave her the cd of her scan & she left.
Once home Gemma could see a full-term baby as clear as day on her scan cd, moving about & looking very healthy.

She couldn't believe it as she had been to her doctor many times complaining of feeling pregnant with negative pregnancy tests. Of course, as Gemma was over forty the doctor didn't bat an eye lid & just told her she was delusional adding he was happy to set her up with a therapist.
Obviously, she ignored this as Gemma wasn't stupid, not by a long shot.

She sadly had some kind of anxiety attack that day at home after seeing her 4D cd with her baby on it as she realised her doctor had been lying to her all along. She was devastated.
It can be very frightening to realise that most (but not all.) of the medical cartel are evil & lying is their native language.

She called an ambulance as she was finding it hard to breathe. At hospital she explained everything & asked the hospital doctors to view her 4D cd but of course they declined so she demanded an X-ray.

The doctors did ask Gemma to take a pregnancy test & being negative they didn't think an X-ray would do any harm as they didn't think for a second, she was pregnant.

During her X-ray she told me she could see the radiologists mouth drop in shock at what he could see on her X-ray – a full term baby – but he soon fixed his expression & told her nothing when she asked what he was seeing.

He just said, "don't worry everything looks normal."

Gemma's story is starting to sound like a missing episode from the XFILES, but it gets worse.

The radiologist seemed to have an attitude when she demanded a copy of her X-ray report.

He said she was not allowed a copy.

I wonder why? Well, they obviously wanted to hide the fact that there was a full-term live baby in her uterus after all because they would be sued for medical negligence at the very least as she had been insisting this was the case for months.

So, still feeling very weak from her anxiety attack she walked the long walk to the hospital admin department, smiled & said simply, "I've just had a routine X-ray & I wonder if I could have a copy for my personal medical records? I'm willing to pay."

The receptionist said this was no problem & not knowing there was a live full-term baby on her X-rays, handed them over without asking for a penny.

Now I have personally seen Gemma's X-ray report & sure enough, there is a full-term baby on it, head down as if it were just waiting for labour to begin.

All any doctor with a brain cell on duty would have to do is LISTEN for a fetal heartbeat & Gemma's baby could be confirmed & she could be induced.
Thankfully, Gemma could afford private medical care so paid to see a specialist obstetrician. After viewing her 4D cd, her X-rays & performing an honest abdominal scan he confirmed that she was thirty-seven weeks pregnant & she went on to have her baby by planned by c section the following week.

It's amazing what money can do.

So, we see again & again that standing up for your medical & human rights during a CP seems to be the ONLY time when standing up for your rights to fair medical treatment is turned against you.

So be wise as serpents & gentle as doves & outsmart the doctors.
This is your human right & the two most important tools of CP psychological warfare you can use on the medical cartel because they have been gas lighting CP women often for years by telling them they are delusional & not pregnant when in fact there is no medical or scientific evidence ANYWHERE that proves unequivocally that all women are only ever pregnant for nine months & even WEBMD, states that a delusional pregnancy can ONLY be confirmed IF a fetal heartbeat has been tested for & NOT FOUND.

It's like saying you have a broken leg just because you fell over & your leg hurts.

Clearly, a doctor has to LOOK for X-ray evidence in order to make a diagnosis of a broken leg.

Of course, this is so obvious it's silly but in the same way, how completely void of thinking capacity a doctor must be to diagnose a false pregnancy in a CP woman without performing all of the relevant diagnostic tests first.

So, if you have been CP for at least nine months & suspect you are full term & your doctor has been less than helpful on many occasions throughout your CP, do NOT go to him for confirmation once your CP has turned normal. There are other medical professionals who can confirm the pregnancy. Now remember, if you suddenly get a positive pregnancy test, even if you tell the medical cartel, you haven't had a cycle for at least five months, they will ALWAYS be looking for a brand-new tiny pregnancy. It's just part of their programming & I can't stress this enough so you must outthink & out smart them.

That kind of new pregnancy is so small that doctors often convince gullible women that they ether can't see a baby, or they can't see a heartbeat, so she needs to use the doctor's drugs ASAP to abort her baby. Even here in the UK this has happened many times, but some women are smart enough to get a second opinion a few weeks later & sure enough their babies are found with a very strong healthy heartbeat.

Come on now. Who are you going to trust? The medical cartel or your own gut? As a True Being you can & must trust your gut as that is the divine spiritual part of you, a part that most humans on the planet today just do not possess as part of their spiritual make up.

I have advised many CP women who feel full term & past nine months CP to handle the medical cartel in the following way once their cycle stops & their pregnancy tests are clearly positive:

1. Go to your local sexual health clinic as they do free pregnancy testing.

2. Remember, if you are over thirty-five take ten years off of your age when filling in the sexual health medical form. They have no link to your medical records in these clinics as they are anonymous.

3. Make it CLEAR to the medical professional that you have been feeling very exhausted & sick for months & you have NOT had a cycle for at last five months, so you took a pregnancy test & it was positive. Tell them you are really hoping that you are NOT pregnant & to be honest, you took so long to take a test because you don't want to be pregnant right now. (This is important, because for some reason I have noticed with the medical cartel that if you tell them the opposite of the result you want, especially with regards to pregnancy, they seem to love confirming what they think you don't want. Plus, it's good to use reverse psychology on them as they have been psychologically abusing CP women for decades.)

4. Once you do your pregnancy test with them & it's positive tell them you need a letter to give to your NEW doctor as you are due to move town in the next few weeks so you will be looking for a new one.

   Make the medical professional write you a letter a. confirming your pregnancy & b. how far along they think you are. (They will probably say you are only about six weeks pregnant as it's just too hard for them to believe you could be five months pregnant or more, especially if you have been a wise CP woman & kept slim throughout your CP.) At this point it's ok to suddenly remember that you put down the wrong age on your form & tell them your correct age & birthday as they have already confirmed the pregnancy.

5. Once you walk out of that sexual health clinic with a letter of pregnancy confirmation rejoice! You are halfway there.

6. Now the next step is very important as if you have a scan right after you have been confirmed by the sexual health clinic, even if it says on the letter, they gave you that they are unsure of how far along you are, the scan tech will always be looking for a NEW pregnancy when in fact you are pregnant with a full-term baby. You cannot trust them to say, "it's a full-term baby!" Yes, there have been many accounts of CP women over the years in newspapers & on tv who didn't know they were pregnant & about to go into labour until they had their first pregnancy scan expecting to see a tiny six-week foetus. (of course, many of these women were true CP women but didn't know because their cycle continued & they didn't think to test.) BUT you just can't rely on your scan tech being that smart or that honest. So, if your letter says it's an early pregnancy, you must WAIT AT LEAST THREE months before your ether pay for a first baby scan, or you can book one through your midwife or doctor. (It might actually be a good idea to change doctors if they have been awful to you during your CP now that you are confirmed.)

7. Now when you finally have your first baby scan at least three months after you have had your positive pregnancy test & conformation at the sexual health clinic, IF they said in the letter, it is an early pregnancy, they will see your CP baby. You see, even if you ARE full term, once they see the baby on the scan, they will almost never think you are more than five or six months pregnant as there is very little difference between a six-month baby in the uterus & a full term baby, all things being considered.

   Not that it's any of their business but if the doctor or tech asks why you have waited so long to get your first scan tell them coolly that you feel that ultrasound waves might be dangerous to the development of a tiny foetus, so you preferred to wait. Which is true in fact.

   Now the above method to get your CP baby found & confirmed once your pregnancy has turned normal (your cycle has stopped & all your pregnancy tests are clearly positive.) is not an exact science but then, nether is most of modern medicine today so you have nothing to lose & everything to gain.

   More importantly this method has worked for many CP women who I have advised all over the world during the last ten years & it worked for me too.

   To illustrate let's observe how Amelia, who we met in chapter seven, used the above steps to have her CP baby finally confirmed once her cycle stopped & her pregnancy tests were clearly positive.

It took almost six weeks of daily, testing, as she was so keen to see her lines get darker, & countless pregnancy tests before Amelia finally felt confident enough to go to the sexual health clinic for pregnancy conformation. At first, she felt annoyed & even guilty at the amount of money she was spending on pregnancy tests each week but what price could she put on finally getting medical confirmation for her CP pregnancy after so many years?

So, on one crisp October morning almost six weeks after she had her first faint positive pregnancy test on an internet cheapie pregnancy test strip, she found herself walking into her local sexual health clinic with quiet confidence.

She filled out her basic details on the paperwork she was given & made sure to take ten years off of her age by putting down thirty-four instead of her real age of forty-four. (Even if you feel silly as you don't look ten years younger doctors are not paid to be rude, so they won't point this out.)

When her name was finally called, she told me that what followed went so smoothly it felt like she was somehow reading from a script because she knew exactly what to say & how to act.

"It was good because if I looked nervous it was because I felt it & this helped to prop up my story.
So, the doctor asked me why I was there & I turned on some drama & said, 'Doctor! I took a pregnancy test a few days ago as I've been feeling so sick & off & well, I'm sorry to say it seems to be positive.' I made sure to look really uncomfortable & confused about this, 'Please, can you tell me that the test is wrong because my career is finally taking off & I really don't think I want a baby right now!'

"The doctor said that home pregnancy tests are normally very reliable but to be sure he would run another pregnancy test.

"Of course, it was positive & the doctor actually seemed sympathetic. He said I had options & asked me how far along I was. I didn't miss a beat & told him that my cycle has been irregular forever, but I did have some spotting around six months ago. I was quite sure from the strong movement that my CP baby was full term, but I knew that I had a tipped uterus, so a full-term baby would be hard to find on a scan unless a doctor was looking for one & I didn't want to push my luck.

"So, I asked the doctor how far along he thought I was. I told him I had a boyfriend but we were on & off so I couldn't be sure on conception dates. I bent the truth & why not? Doctors have been lying to CP women since forever. He asked if he could feel my belly & when he did, he said he thought I might be in my second trimester, which was a result as at least he didn't say I was only six weeks pregnant!

"Finally, it was time for me to go for the money shot so I said, 'doctor I am due to move town in two weeks so I will have to change doctors. Will you please give me a note or a letter I can give to my new GP confirming the pregnancy & how far along you think I am? I can then discuss all of my options with my new GP right away.'

"The doctor said yes of course & hurriedly scribbled a letter. As he handed it to me & I went to leave I tried to squash the smile that was creeping over my face, thanked him & holding the letter close to my chest got the hell out of there!

I walked a few short feet from the clinic, tore the letter open & read:

To whom it may concern,

This is a letter of pregnancy confirmation for Amelia Lewis as she has had a positive pregnancy test today at the sexual health clinic. Patient is not sure of her dates & suffers from irregular cycles but

from examination appears to be in her second trimester, so twenty to twenty-six weeks as the uterus is high....

"I was shaking & smiling; I was so dizzy with relief Neo! After all these years of confusion, pain & shame I finally had my pregnancy confirmation from a doctor! It felt unreal but I knew that finally, because my pregnancy was real to the doctors, I would be holding my CP baby for sure in a matter of months!"

Amelia went on to call & book a private fetal scan for the following day & by teatime had finally seen her baby on a scan, found out she was having a baby boy who was extremely healthy, been given a due date & been told that she was six months pregnant.

And all because of her precious doctor's letter of pregnancy confirmation. Something she may not have thought to ask for if she hadn't had access to the advice in this chapter on how to deal with the medical cartel once a CP turns normal.

All except one of my children were CP but with the eldest I didn't know because my cycle continued & I didn't think to test. I could often feel a lot of fast painful movement in my belly specially if I bent down too quickly to pick something up, so looking back it all made sense.

When my cycle finally stopped & my pregnancy test was positive, I believed it was a new pregnancy & so did my doctor but that was fine as back then you didn't have a first scan until you were around four months pregnant. I had my first scan at sixteen weeks & although the baby was measuring a little ahead of dates as it had been a CP baby, the doctors saw nothing strange about this.

So, in summary to get your baby confirmed if you are at last nine months CP once your CP turns normal: go to the sexual health clinic to have a pregnancy test once your home pregnancy tests are showing strong big fat positives.

Make sure to tell them you have just taken a pregnancy test, it's positive but you're hoping they can tell you it's wrong, you haven't had a cycle for around five months & you have been feeling sick & exhausted for a while.

Get a letter of pregnancy confirmation from the sexual health clinic & ask them to write on the letter how far along they think you are.

WAIT for three months before you have your first baby scan IF they wrote in the letter that it's a new pregnancy but be led your intuition. You may feel your baby will be safely found if you go for the scan sooner or even later. Once your baby is found on ultrasound enjoy the rest of your pregnancy however far along the doctors say you are & no matter how long you have been CP because your nightmare is OVER!

In chapter one of Principles of mathematics Bertrand Russel reveals, ". mathematical reasoning is not strictly formal but always uses intuitions, i.e... a priori knowledge of space & time.

The ideas in this book are both logical & intuitive, but the take home theory is that a woman going through a cryptic pregnancy, i.e.: a woman who feels she is pregnant despite negative pregnancy tests, can be freed from the false stigma & assumption that she is having a delusional pregnancy by simply using The Finger Pulse & Doppler Test & confirming that there is a second heartbeat on the doppler of 120bpm or more, whilst hers taken at the same time on a finger pulse is 60 to 90bpm, if she is truly pregnant.
As no woman alive in this world has ever been found to have two separate heartbeats inside of her body unless she is pregnant.

Bibliography

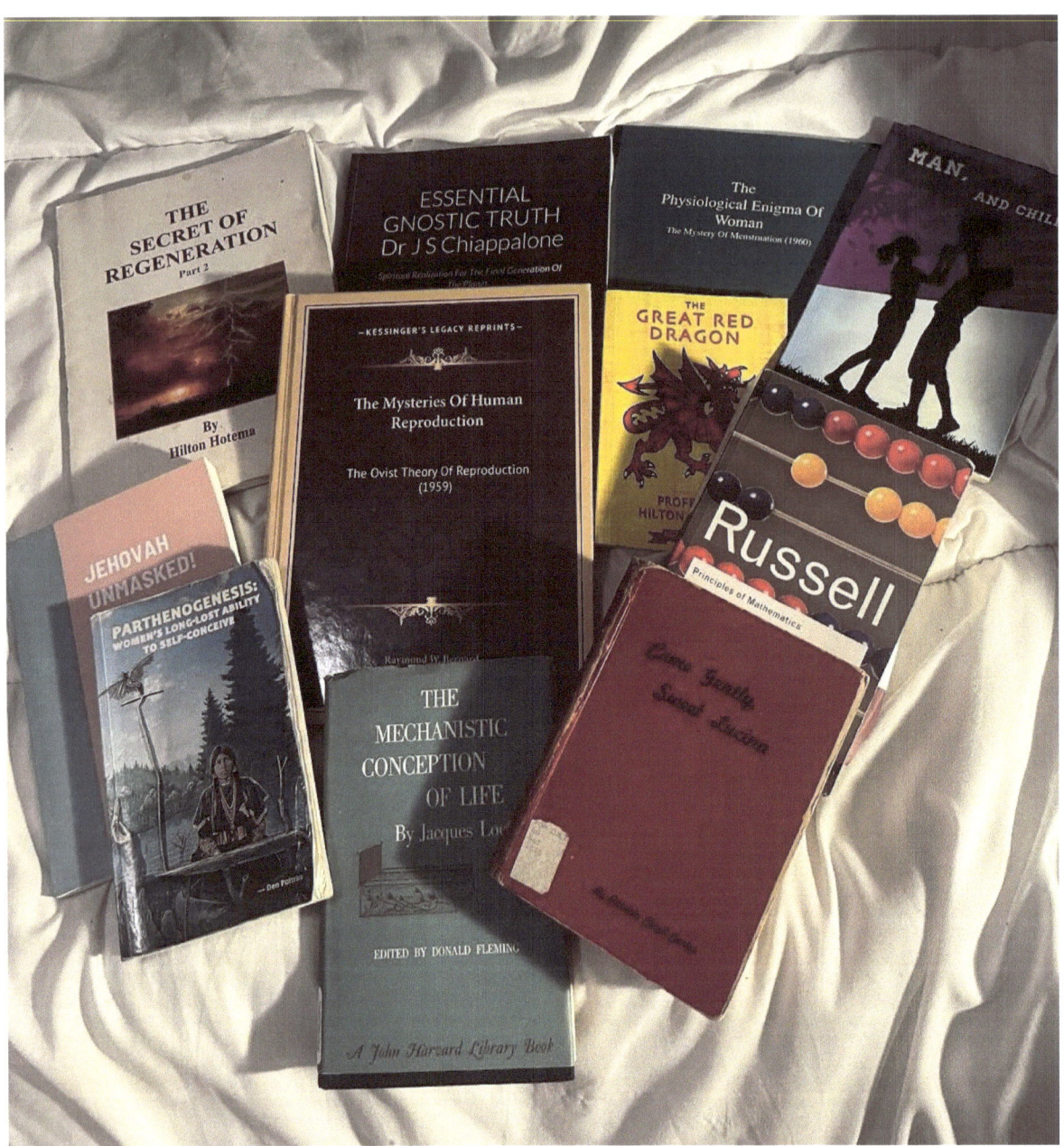

www.ingramcontent.com/pod-product-compliance
Lightning Source LLC
Chambersburg PA
CBHW051159220526

45473CB00003B/831